Textbook of Microbiology for Health Sciences

Textbook of Microbiology for Health Sciences

Mathew George
Director Holy Queen college of pharmaceutical
sciences and research Thrissur
Kerala.

Lincy Joseph
Academic Director Holy Queen college of pharmaceutical
sciences and research Thrissur
Kerala.

PharmaMed Press
An Imprint of BSP Books Pvt. Ltd.
4-4-309/316, Giriraj Lane,
Sultan Bazar, Hyderabad - 500 095.

Textbook of Microbiology for Health Sciences

by **Mathew George, Lincy Joseph**

Published by

PharmaMed Press

An Imprint of BSP Books Pvt. Ltd.

4-4-309/316, Giriraj Lane, Sultan Bazar, Hyderabad - 500 095.

Phone: 040-23445688; Fax: 91+40-23445611

E-mail: info@pharmamedpress.com

www.pharmamedpress.com/pharmamedpress.net

ISBN: 978-93-48734-12-9 (Hardback)

Foreward

I am extremely happy to write foreword on "**Textbook of Microbiology for Health Sciences**" jointly written by **Prof. Dr. Mathew George, Director and Prof. Dr. Lincy Joseph, Academic Director – Holy Queen College of Pharmaceutical Sciences & Research –Thrissur, Kerala**. who have been taken the task of writing the Textbook for Microbiology.

Dr. M. George & Dr. L. Joseph both done **Post Docs (From USA)**, and both have many **Granted Patents** to their credit. I am sure that teaching faculty at every Point and stage of their career will enrich and strengthen their knowledge by discussion – leading pattern and practices presented in this text book. This textbook is a guide for Medical, Dental, Pharmacy, & Nursing students… etc.

This textbook contains detailed information of Microbiology and has rendered valuable service to the Profession of health sciences.

I take this opportunity to encourage the authors for their efforts and expecting more such efforts.

Prof. Dr. MD Karvekar

Former Executive Committee Member,

PCI - New Delhi

Preface

This book is the first edition and first attempt to write "Textbook of Microbiology for Health Sciences." It is focused on studying microbiology for Health Sciences and Allied Health Sciences student community. In the multidisciplinary healthcare system, healthcare practitioners need to have in depth knowledge of Microbiology. All the topics are presented in a simplified manner.

The scope of the book is to impart basic knowledge in Microbiology for health and allied health sciences students. The following topics are dealt with here:

Introduction, history of microbiology, its branches, scope, and its importance. Introduction to Prokaryotes and Eukaryotes. Study of ultrastructure and morphological classification of bacteria, nutritional requirements, raw materials used for culture media, and physical parameters for growth. Growth curve, isolation, and preservation methods for pure cultures. Cultivation of anaerobes, quantitative measurement of bacterial growth (total & viable count). Study of different types of phase contrast microscopy, dark field microscopy, and electron microscopy.

Identification of bacteria using staining techniques (simple, Gram's & Acid-fast staining) and biochemical tests (IMViC). Study of principle, procedure, merits, demerits, and applications of physical, chemical, gaseous, radiation, and mechanical methods of sterilization. Evaluation of the efficiency of sterilization methods. Equipment employed in large-scale sterilization, sterility indicators.

Study of morphology, classification, reproduction/replication, and cultivation of fungi and viruses. Classification and mode of action of disinfectants. Factors influencing disinfection, antiseptics, and their evaluation for bacteriostatic and bactericidal actions. Evaluation of bactericidal & bacteriostatic actions. Sterility testing of products (solids, liquids, ophthalmic, and other sterile products) according to various pharmacopoeias.

Designing of aseptic area, laminar flow equipment, study of different sources of contamination in an aseptic area, and methods of prevention, clean area classification. Principles and methods of different microbiological assays. Methods for standardization of antibiotics, vitamins, and amino acids. Assessment of a new antibiotic.

Types of spoilage, factors affecting the microbial spoilage of pharmaceutical products, sources and types of microbial contaminants, and assessment of microbial contamination and spoilage. Preservation of pharmaceutical products using antimicrobial agents, evaluation of microbial stability of formulations. Growth of animal cells in culture, general procedure for cell culture, primary, established, and transformed cell cultures. Application of cell cultures in the pharmaceutical industry and research.

It is a great privilege to render this book. Thanks to all readers of this book and sincerely accept all constructive criticism and valuable comments to incorporate genuine points in the upcoming edition. Hope this textbook will be fruitful for the students.

Authors-

Contents

UNIT I

Bacteria and it's Cultivation

Microbiology

Microbiology is the study of Microbes which are generally too small needed magnification to see. These microbes include viruses, bacteria, algae, fungi and protozoa. Microorganisms /Microbes are the living organisms that are less than 1 milli meter in diameter can exist as single cells or clusters.

Microbiology is the branch of Life Science and it can be applied or basic. Microbiology is linked to many other scientific disciplines including biochemistry, cell biology, evolution, ecology.

Branches of Microbiology

By Taxonomy

Bacteriology: the study of bacteria.

Immunology: the study of the immune system. It looks at the relationships between pathogens such as bacteria and viruses and their hosts.

Mycology: the study of fungi, such as yeasts and moulds.

Nematology: the study of nematodes (roundworms).

Parasitology: the study of parasites. Not all parasites are microorganisms, but many are. Protozoa and bacteria can be parasitic; the study of bacterial parasites is usually categorized as part of bacteriology.

Phycology: the study of algae.

Protozoology: the study of protozoa, single-celled organisms like amoebae.

Virology: the study of viruses.

SCOPE OF MICROBIOLOGY

Microorganisms are recognized as the basicresearch tools as they help to understand the chemical and physical basis of life as they are the dominant group of living organisms in the biosphere and are actively involved in our day to day activities. Microbiology primarily paves way to analyse the biochemical and genetic background of living things. Moreover, as microbes are the excellent models for understanding the cell functions and as they play important role in the field of medicine,

agriculture and industry that assures human welfare, microbiology is considered as one of thevital branch of science with utmost promising scopes.

By focussed **on application** microbiology can be divided as mentioned below; Eg;

***Agricultural microbiology*:** the study of microorganisms that interact with plants and soils.

***Food microbiology*:** the study of microorganisms that spoil food or cause foodborne illnesses. Can also study how microorganisms are used in food production, such as fermentation of beer.

***Medical microbiology*:** the study of microorganisms responsible for human disease.

***Microbial biotechnology*:** using microbes in industrial or consumer products.

***Pharmaceutical microbiology*:** the study of microorganisms used in pharmaceutical products, such as vaccines and antibiotics.

Little History/Background of Microbiology

The theory of biogenesis proposes that new living organisms can be created only from other previously existing living organisms as a result of sexual or asexual reproduction. Spontaneous generation or abiogenesis is the exact opposite of biogenesis stating that life can come from non-living.

Antonie van Leeuwenhoek (1632–1723) was one of the first people to observe microorganisms, using a microscope. He reported on the ubiquity of microbes. Louis Pasteur performed several experiments to demonstrate that microbial life does not arise spontaneously. Robert Koch (1843–1910) established that microbes can cause disease. Robert Koch isolated the bacteria which cause anthrax and tuberculosis. Koch's four postulates are 1) The microorganism must be found in diseased but should not be found in healthy organisms. 2) The microorganism must be cultured from the diseased individual and should be cultured in pure culture. 3) The cultured microorganism should cause disease when introduced into a healthy organism. 4) The microorganism re-isolated from the inoculated, diseased individual and should be matched to the original microorganism.

The twentieth century saw numerous advances in bacteriology, indicating their diversity, ancient lineage, and general importance. Most notably, a number of scientists around the world made contributions to the field of microbial ecology, showing that bacteria were essential to food webs and for the overall health of the Earth's ecosystems. The discovery that some bacteria produced compounds lethal to other bacteria led to the development of antibiotics, which revolutionized the field of medicine.

Prokaryotes & Eukaryotes

Based on the structure of nucleus, fundamentally two types of cells exist. They are

i. Prokaryotes and **ii.** Eukaryotes

Prokaryotes have a relatively simple morphology and lack a true membrane-delimited nucleus. All bacteria and archaea are prokaryotic. ARCHAEA are phylogenetically related prokaryotes that are distinguished from bacteria by many features, most notably-Bacteria contain peptidoglycan in the cell wall; archaea do not. The cell membrane in bacteria is a lipid bilayer; in archaea, it can be a lipid bilayer or a monolayer. Eg for Archaea: Methanobacterium which generate methane gas.

Prokaryote is a Greek word, pro - before and karyon – nucleus.

Eucaryotes are morphologically complex and have a true, membrane-enclosed nucleus eg: Algae, fungi, protozoa.

Eukaryote is a Greek word, eu - true.

DIFFERENCE BETWEEN PROKARYOTES AND EUKARYOTES

Sl. No	Characteristics	Prokaryotic	Eukaryotic
1	Cell Size	Generally, 1 to 10 μm in linear dimension	Generally, 5 to 100 μm inlinear dimension
2	Cell division	Binary fission	Mitosis
3	Cellular organism	Unicellular	Mostly multicellular withdifferentiation of manytypes.
4	Cell wall	Complex structure with peptidoglycan layer, proteinand lipids	Absent or composed of cellulose or chitin
5	Plasma membrane	Present, no sterols except inmycoplasma	Present, contain sterols
6	Metabolism	Anaerobic or	Aerobic

Table Contd...

		aerobic	
7	DNA	Circular DNA in cytoplasm.	Very long, linear DNA molecule bounded by nuclear envelope
8	Membrane bound Nucleus	Absent	Present.
9	Extra chromosomal DNA	Present	Absent
10	Histones	Absent	Present
11	Membrane bound organelles	Absent	Present (Nucleus, mitochondria, chloroplast, ER
12	Ribosomes	70S type	80S type
13	Lysosomes	Absent	Present
14	Locomotion	Rotating flagella and glidingmovement	Undulating flagella &ciliaand amoeboid movement
15	Flagella	Consists of two protein building blocks	Consists of multiple Microtubules
16	Pili	Present	Absent
17	Site for cellular respiration	Cell membrane	Mitochondria
18	Examples	Bacteria and Archaea	Fungi, Algae and Protozoa

Bacteria

Bacteria (singular: bacterium) are classified as prokaryotes, which are single-celled organisms with a simple internal structure that lacks a nucleus, and contains DNA that either floats freely in a twisted, thread-like mass called the nucleoid, or in separate, circular pieces called plasmids.

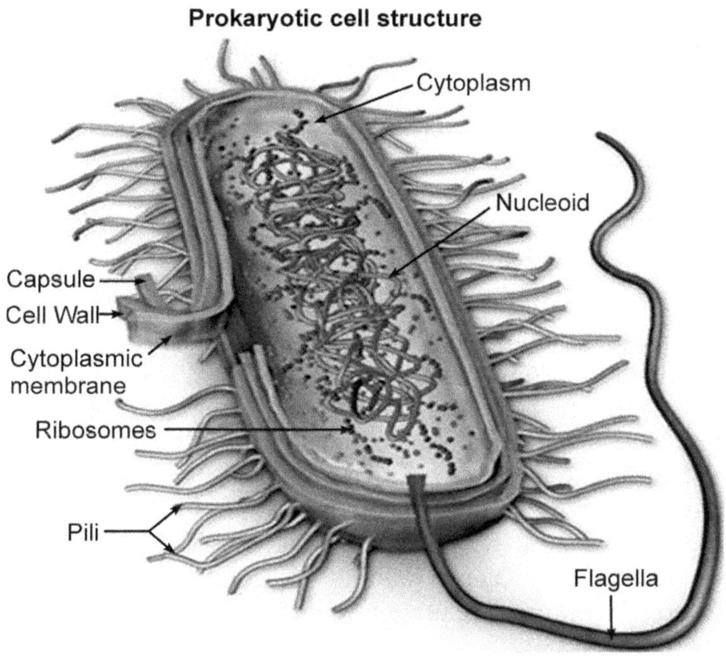

Fig 1.1. Prokaryotic Cell Structure.

For example, one species that lives symbiotically in the large intestine manufacture's vitamin K, an essential blood clotting factor. Other species are beneficial indirectly. Bacteria give yogurt its tangy flavour and sourdough bread its sour taste. They make it possible for ruminant animals (cows, sheep, goats) to digest plant cellulose and for some plants, (soybean, peas, alfalfa) to convert nitrogen to a more usable form.

Cell Envelope - The cell envelope is made up of two to three layers: the interior cytoplasmic membrane, the cell wall, and in some species of bacteria an outer capsule.

Capsule - It is an outer protective covering found in bacterial cells, in addition to cell wall. It helps in moisture retention and help in attachment of cells to absorb nutrients.

Cell Wall - Each bacterium is enclosed by a rigid cell wall composed of peptidoglycan, a protein-sugar (polysaccharide) molecule. The wall gives the cell its shape and surrounds the cytoplasmic membrane, protecting it from the environment. It also helps to anchor appendages like the pili and flagella, which originate in the cytoplasm membrane and protrude through the wall to the outside. The strength of the wall is responsible for keeping the cell from bursting when there are large differences in osmotic pressure between the cytoplasm and the environment.

Cytoplasm - The cytoplasm, or protoplasm, of bacterial cells is where the functions for cell growth, metabolism, and replication are carried out. It is a gel-like matrix composed of water, enzymes, nutrients, wastes, and gases and contains cell structures such as ribosomes, a chromosome, and plasmids. The cell envelope encases the cytoplasm and all its components. Unlike the eukaryotic (true) cells, bacteria do not have a membrane enclosed nucleus. The chromosome, a single, continuous strand of DNA, is localized, but not contained, in a region of the cell called the nucleoid. All the other cellular components are scattered throughout the cytoplasm.

One of those components, **plasmids,** are small, extrachromosomal genetic structures carried by many strains of bacteria. Like the chromosome, plasmids are made of a circular piece of DNA. Unlike the chromosome, they are not involved in reproduction. Only the chromosome has the genetic instructions for initiating and carrying out cell division, or binary fission, the primary means of reproduction in bacteria. Plasmids replicate independently of the chromosome and, while not essential for survival, appear to give bacteria a selective advantage. While in the case of virus which encase their genetic material in a protective protein coat called a capsid.

Plasmids are passed on to other bacteria through two means. For most plasmid types, copies in the cytoplasm are passed on to daughter cells during binary fission. Other types of plasmids, however, form a tubelike structure at the surface called a pilus that passes copies of the plasmid to other bacteria during conjugation, a process by which bacteria exchange genetic information. Plasmids have been shown to be instrumental in the transmission of special properties, such as antibiotic drug resistance, resistance to heavy metals, and virulence factors necessary for infection of animal or plant hosts.

Cytoplasmic Membrane - A layer of phospholipids and proteins, called the cytoplasmic membrane, encloses the interior of the bacterium, regulating the flow of materials in and out of the cell.

Flagella - Flagella (singular, flagellum) are hair like structures or organelles provide locomotion to bacteria. Flagella have three parts namely basal body, hook and filament. The basal body consists of a rod and a series of rings which are attached to the cell wall and the cytoplasmic membrane. The rings which are basically proteins. There are three types of rings, namely the L-ring attached to the lipopolysaccharide, the P-ring attached to the peptidoglycan layer, and the M-S ring which is attached to the cytoplasmic membrane.

The hook is a flexible link between filament and the basal body proteins. The filament is a rigid, helical structure that extends from the cell surface.

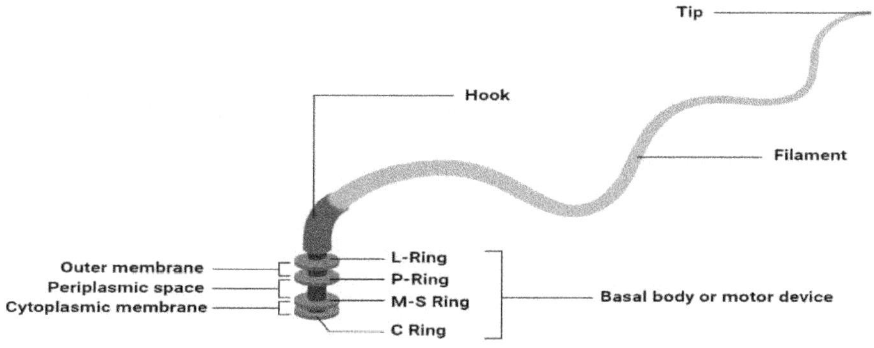

Structure of Flagellum of Gram Negative Bacterium

A single flagellum at one end or the other is called monotrichous. They can be found at either or both ends of a bacterium (lophotrichous) or all over its surface (peritrichous). The flagella beat in a propeller-like motion to help the bacterium move toward nutrients; away from toxic chemicals; or, in the case of the photosynthetic cyanobacteria; toward the light.

Nucleoid - The nucleoid is a region of cytoplasm where the chromosomal DNA is located. It is not a membrane bound nucleus, but simply an area of the cytoplasm where the strands of DNA are found. Most bacteria have a single, circular chromosome that is responsible for replication, although a few species do have two or more. Smaller circular auxiliary DNA strands, called plasmids, are also found in the cytoplasm.

Pili - Many species of bacteria have pili (singular, pilus), small hairlike projections emerging from the outside cell surface. These outgrowths assist the bacteria in attaching to other cells and surfaces, such as teeth, intestines, and rocks. Without pili, many disease-causing bacteria lose their ability to infect because they're unable to attach to host tissue. Specialized pili are used for conjugation, during which two bacteria exchange fragments of plasmid DNA.

Ribosomes - Ribosomes are microscopic "factories" found in all cells, including bacteria. They translate the genetic code from the molecular language of nucleic acid to that of amino acids—the building blocks of proteins. Proteins are the molecules that perform all the functions of cells and living organisms.

Morphological classification

Bacteria can be classified into **six** major groups on morphological basis.

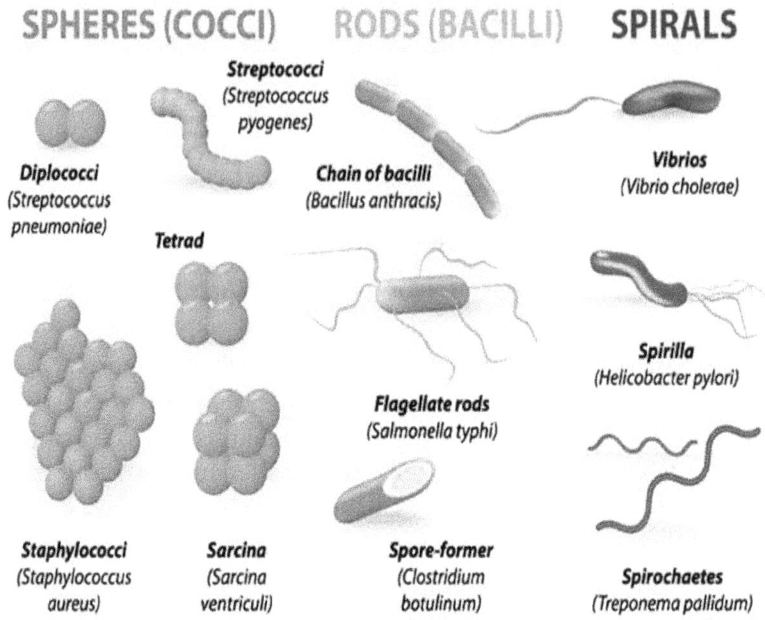

Fig 1.2. Classification of bacteria based on morphology.

1. **TRUE BACTERIA** – Cocci. These are spherical or oval cells. On the basis of arrangement of individual organisms, they can be described as – Monococci (Cocci in singles) – Monococcus species, Diplococci (Cocci in pairs) – Streptococcus pneumoniae, Staphylococci (Cocci in grape-like clusters) – Staphylococcus aureus, Streptococci (Cocci in chains) – Streptococcus pyogenes, Tetrad (Cocci in group of four) - Micrococcus species, Sarcina (Cocci in group of eight) Bacilli– These are rod-shaped bacteria.

2. **ACTINOMYCETES** (actin - ray, mykes-fungus) (actin - ray) These are rigid organisms like true bacteria but they resemble fungi in that they exhibit branching and tend to form filaments. They are termed such because of their resemblance to sun rays when seen in tissue sections.

3. **SPIROCHAETES** These are relatively longer, slender, non-branched microorganisms of spiral shape having several coils.

4. **MYCOPLASMAS** These bacteria lack in rigid cell wall (cell wall lacking) and are highly pleomorphic and of indefinite shape. They occur in round or oval bodies and in interlacing filaments.

5. **RICKETTSIAE AND CHLAMYDIAE** These are very small, obligate parasites, and at one time were considered closely related to the viruses.

Classification on the basis of Gram Stain and Bacterial Cell Wall

It allows a large proportion of clinically important bacteria to be classified as either Gram positive or negative based on their morphology and differential staining properties. Slides are sequentially stained with crystal violet, iodine, then distained with alcohol and counter-stained with safranin. Gram positive bacteria stain blue-purple and Gram-negative bacteria stain red.

Classification of Bacteria on the Basis of Mode of Nutrition

Phototrophs: These bacteria gain energy from light. Phototrophs are further divided into two groups on the basis of source of electron.

Photolithotrophs: These bacteria gain energy from light and ***uses reduced inorganic compounds*** such as H_2S as clectron sourcc. Photo organotrophs: These bacteria gain energy from light and ***uses organic compounds*** such as succinate as electron source.

Chemotrophs: Those bacteria gain energy from chemical compounds. Chemotrophs are further divided into two groups on the basis of source of electron.

Chemolithotrophs: These gain energy from oxidation of chemical compound and reduces inorganic compounds such as NH_3 as electron source. Eg. Nitrosomonas.

Chemoorganotrophs: These gain energy from chemical compounds and uses organic compound such as glucose and amino acids as source of electron. Eg. Pseudomonas pseudoflava.

Autotrophs: Those bacteria which uses carbondioxide as sole source of carbon to prepare its own food. Autotrophs are divided into two types on the basis of energy utilized to assimilate carbondioxide i.e., Photoautotrophs and chemoautotrophs.

Photoautotrophs: These utilized light to assimilate CO_2. Chemoautotrophs: These utilize chemical energy to assimilate CO_2.

Heterotrophs: Those bacteria which uses organic compound as carbon source. They lack the ability to fix CO_2. Most of the human pathogenic bacteria are heterotrophic in nature.

Classification of Bacteria on Basis of Temperature Requirement

major types on the basis of their temperatures response as indicated below:

a. **Psychrophiles**: Bacteria that can grow at 0°Cor below but the optimum temperature of growth is 15 °C or below and maximum temperature is 20°C are called psychrophiles.

Examples: Vibrio psychroerythrus, vibrio marinus, Psychroflexus.

b. **Psychrotrops** (facultative psychrophiles):

Those bacteria that can grow even at 0°C but optimum temperature for growth is (20-30)°C. Eg: Pseudomonas fluorescens, Micrococcus.

c. **Mesophiles:**

Those bacteria that can grow best between (25-40) °C but optimum temperature for growth is 37^0C, most of the human pathogens are mesophilic in nature.

Examples: E. coli, Salmonella, Klebsiella, Staphylococci.

d. **Thermophiles:** Those bacteria that can best grow above 45°C.

Examples: Streptococcus thermophiles, Bacillus stearothermophilus, Thermus aquaticus.

e. **Hypethermophiles:**

Those bacteria that have optimum temperature of growth above 80^0C.

Mostly Archeobacteria are hyperthermophiles.

Examples: Thermodesulfobacterium, Aquifex, Pyrolobus fumari,

Classification of Bacteria on the Basis of Oxygen Requirement

Obligate Aerobes: Require oxygen to live.

Example: Pseudomonas, common nosocomial pathogen.

Facultative Anaerobes: Can use oxygen, but can grow in its absence.

They have complex set of enzymes. Most bacteria of medical importance arefacultative anaerobes.

Examples: E. coli, Staphylococcus, yeasts, & many intestinal bacteria.

Obligate Anaerobes:

Cannot use oxygen and are harmed by the presence of toxic forms of oxygen.

Examples: Clostridium bacteria that cause tetanus and botulism.

Aerotolerant Anaerobes: Cannot use oxygen, but tolerate its presence. Can break down toxic forms of oxygen.

Examples: Lactobacillus carries out fermentation regardless of oxygen presence.

Microaerophiles: Require oxygen, but at low concentrations. Sensitive to toxic forms of oxygen. Eg: Campylobacter.

Classification of Bacteria on the Basis of pH of Growth

Acidophiles: These bacteria grow best at an acidic pH. The cytoplasm of these bacteria is acidic in nature. Some acidopiles are thermophilic in nature, such bacteria are called Thermoacidophiles.

Example: Thiobacillus thioxidans, Thiobacillus, ferroxidans, Sulfolobus

Alkaliphiles: These bacteria grow best at an alkaline pH.

Example: Vibrio cholerae optimum pH of growth is 8.2.

Neutrophiles: These bacteria grow best at neutral pH (6.5-7.5).

Example: E. coli

Classification of Bacteria on the Basis of Osmotic Pressure Requirement

Halophiles: Require moderate to large salt concentrations.

Cell membrane of halophilic bacteria is made up of glycoprotein with high content of negatively charged glutamic acid and aspartic acids. So high concentration of $Na+$ ion concentration is required to shield the –ve charge. Ocean water contains 3.5% salt. Most such bacteria are present in the oceans.

Archeobacteria, Halobacterium, Halococcus.

Extreme or Obligate Halophiles: Require a very high salt concentration (20 to 30%). Bacteria in Dead Sea.

Facultative Halophiles: Do not require high salt concentrations for growth, but tolerate up to 2% salt or more.

Classification of Bacteria on the Basis of Number of Flagella

Atrichos: These bacteria have no flagella. **Example:** Corynebacterium diptherae.

Monotrichous: One flagellum is attached to one end of the bacteria cell. **Example:** Vibro cholerae.

Lophotrichous: Bunch of flagella is attached to one end of the bacteria cell. **Example:** Pseudomonas.

Amphitrichous: Bunch of flagella arising from both end of the bacteria cell. **Example:** Rhodospirillum rubrum.

Peritrichous: The flagella are evenly distributed surrounding the entire bacterial cell. **Example:** Bacillus.

Classification of Bacteria on the basis of Spore Formation

1) Spore forming bacteria: Those bacteria that produce spore during unfavourable condition.

These are further divided into two groups:

i) ***Endospore forming bacteria*:** Spore is produced within the bacterial cell. **Examples:** Bacillus, Clostridium, Sporosarcina etc

ii) ***Exospore forming bacteria:*** Spore is produced outside the cell.

Example: Methylosinus

2) ***Non-sporing bacteria:***

Those bacteria which do not produce spores.

Example: E. coli, Salmonella.

Nutritional Requirements

The bacterial cell contains water (80% of total weight), proteins, polysaccharides, lipids, nucleic acids, mucopeptides and low molecular weight compounds.

For growth and nutrition of bacteria, the minimum nutritional requirements are water, a source of carbon, a source of nitrogen and some inorganic salts. Water is the vehicle of entry of all nutrients into the cell and for the elimination of waste products.

Their nutritional requirements vary widely. Some may require only a single organic substance like glucose. Others may need a large number of different compounds like amino acids, nucleotides, lipids, carbohydrates and coenzymes. Bacteria require a supply of inorganic salts. They require anions like phosphate and sulphate anions and cations like sodium, potassium, magnesium, iron and calcium. Some ions like cobalt may be required in trace amounts. Some bacteria require certain organic compounds in minute quantities. These are called growth factors or bacterial vitamins. Growth factors are called essential when growth does not occur in their absence. Accessory growth factors are those which enhance growth without being absolutely necessary for it. In many cases, bacterial vitamins are same as vitamins necessary for nutrition of mammals, for example, B group vitamins – thiamine, riboflavin, pyridoxine, nicotinic acid, folic acid and vitamin B12.

Gaseous Requirements: Depending on the influence of oxygen on growth and survival, bacteria are divided into **aerobes** and a**naerobes**. Aerobic bacteria require oxygen for growth. They may be ***obligate aerobes*** or *facultative anaerobe*s. Obligate aerobes grow only in the presence of oxygen, for eg. Cholera bacillus. Facultative anaerobes are ordinarily aerobic but can grow in the absence of oxygen, though less abundantly. Anaerobic bacteria, such as clostridia grow in the absence of oxygen. Obligate anaerobes may even die on exposure to oxygen. Microaerophilic bacteria are those that grow best in the presence of low oxygen tension.

In case of aerobes, atmospheric oxygen is the final electron acceptor in the process of respiration (aerobic respiration). In this case, the carbon and energy source may be completely oxidised to carbon dioxide and water. Energy is provided by the production of energy-rich phosphate bonds and the conversion of adenosine diphosphate (ADP) to adenosine triphosphate (ATP). This process is called ***oxidative phosphorylation***. Anaerobic bacteria use compounds like nitrates or sulphates instead of oxygen as final electron acceptors in the process of respiration (anaerobic respiration). A more common process used by these bacteria in anaerobic metabolism is ***fermentation.*** It is defined as the process by which complex organic compounds, such as glucose, are broken down by the action of enzymes into simpler compounds without the use of oxygen. This process leads to the formation of several organic end products such as organic acids and alcohols, as well as of gas (carbon dioxide and hydrogen). For example, Escherichia coli ferments glucose with the production of acid and gas. It also ferments lactose. During the process of fermentation, energy-rich phosphate bonds are produced by the introduction of organic phosphate into intermediate metabolites. This process is known as ***substrate-level phosphorylation***. The energy-rich phosphate groups so formed are used for conversion of ADP to ATP. All bacteria require some amounts of carbon dioxide for growth. This is obtained from the atmosphere or from the cellular metabolism of the bacterial cell. Some bacteria like Brucella abortus require much higher levels of carbon dioxide (5- 10%) for growth. They are called capnophilic.

Temperature Requirements: Bacteria vary in their requirement of temperature for growth. The temperature at which growth occurs best is known as the "***optimum temperature***". In the case of most pathogenic bacteria, the optimum temperature is 37°C. Bacteria which grow best at temperatures of 25-40°C are called ***mesophilic***, for example Escherichia coli. Psychrophilic bacteria are those that grow best at temperatures below 20°C. They are soil and water saprophytes and may cause spoilage of refrigerated food. ***Thermophilic bacteria*** are those which grow best at high temperatures, 55-80°C. They may cause spoilage of under processed canned food. Some thermophiles, for example Geobacillus stearothermophilus, form spores that are highly thermoresistant.

The Effect of pH on Growth

The pH, or hydrogen ion concentration, $[H^+]$, of natural environments varies from about 0.5 in the most acidic soils to about 10.5 in the most alkaline lakes. The range of pH over which an organism grows is defined by **three cardinal points**: the **minimum pH**, below which the organism cannot grow, the **maximum pH**, above which the organism cannot grow, and the **optimum pH**, at which the organism grows best.

Microorganisms which grow at an optimum pH well below neutrality (7.0) are called **acidophiles.** Those which grow best at neutral pH are called **neutrophiles** and those that grow best under alkaline conditions are called **alkaliphiles.**

In the construction and use of culture media, one must always consider the optimum pH for growth of a desired organism and incorporate buffers in order to maintain the pH of the medium in the changing milieu of bacterial waste products that accumulate during growth. Many pathogenic bacteria exhibit a relatively narrow range of pH over which they will grow. Most diagnostic media for the growth and identification of human pathogens have a pH near 7.

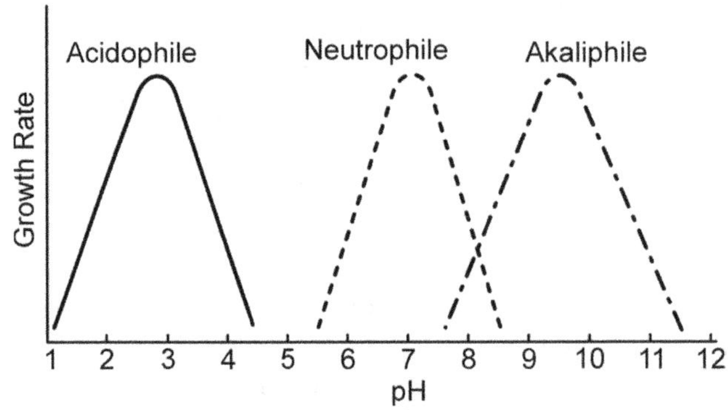

Fig 1.3. Growth rate vs pH for three environmental classes of procaryotes. Most free-living bacteria grow over a pH range of about three units. Note the symmetry of the curves below and above the optimum pH.

Trace Elements

Trace elements are metal ions required by certain cells in such small amounts that it is difficult to detect (measure) them, and it is not necessary to add them to culture media as nutrients. The usual cations that qualify as trace elements in bacterial nutrition are Mn, Co, Zn, Cu, and Mo.

Culture Media for the Growth of Bacteria

For any bacterium to be propagated for any purpose it is necessary to provide the appropriate biochemical and biophysical environment. The biochemical (nutritional) environment is made available as a **culture medium**, and depending upon the special needs of particular bacteria (as well as particular investigators) a large variety and types of culture media have been developed with different purposes and uses. Culture Medium is defined as Nutrient material prepared for microbial growth in the laboratory. Requirements: Must be sterile & contain appropriate nutrients. Must be incubated at appropriate temperature.

Culture media are employed in the isolation and maintenance of pure cultures of bacteria and are also used for identification of bacteria according to their biochemical and physiological properties. Culture is defined as microbes that grow and multiply in or on a culture medium.

Media Can be used to-Enrich the numbers of bacteria, select for certain bacteria and suppress others, Differentiate among different kinds of bacteria.

The manner in which bacteria are cultivated, and the purpose of culture media, varies widely. **Liquid media** are used for growth of pure batch cultures, while solidified media are used widely for the isolation of pure cultures, for estimating viable bacterial populations, and a variety of other purposes. The usual gelling agent for solid or **semisolid medium** is **agar**, a hydrocolloid derived from red algae. Agar is used because of its unique physical properties (it melts at 100°C and remains liquid until cooled to 40°C, the temperature at which it gels) and because it cannot be metabolized by most bacteria. Hence as a medium component it is relatively inert; it simply holds (gels) nutrients that are in aqueous solution.

BASIC REQUIREMENTS OF CULTURE MEDIA

1 **Nutrients:** proteins/peptides/amino-acids.

2 **Energy**: carbohydrates.

3 **Essential metals and minerals:** calcium, magnesium, iron, trace metals: phosphates, sulphates etc.

4 **Buffering agents:** phosphates, acetates etc.

5 **Indicators for pH change:** phenol red, bromo-cresol purple etc.

6 **Selective agents**: chemicals, antimicrobial agents.

7 **Gelling agent:** usually agar.

1 **Classification of bacterial culture media on the basis of consistency**

 1 Solid medium

 2 Semisolid medium

 3 Liquid (Broth) medium

2 **Classification of Bacterial Culture media on the basis of purpose/ functional use/ application**

 1 General-purpose media/ Basic media

 2 Enriched medium (Added growth factors):

 3 Selective and enrichment media

  a. Selective medium

  b. Enrichment culture medium

4 Differential/ indicator medium: differential appearance:
5 Transport media
6 Anaerobic media:
7 Assay media

Solid medium

Solid medium contains agar at a concentration of 1.5-2.0% or some other, mostly inert solidifying agent. Solid medium has physical structure and allows bacteria to grow in physically informative or useful ways (e.g. as colonies or in streaks). Solid medium is useful *for **isolating bacteria*** or for determining the colony characteristics of the isolate.

Semisolid medium

Semisolid medium is prepared with agar at concentrations of 0.5% or less. Semisolid medium has a soft custard-like consistency and is useful for the cultivation of microaerophilic bacteria or for the determination of bacterial motility.

Liquid (Broth) medium

These media contain specific amounts of nutrients but don't have a trace of gelling agents such as gelatin or agar. Broth medium serves various purposes such as propagation of a large number of organisms, fermentation studies, and various other tests. e.g. sugar fermentation tests, MR-VR broth

General-purpose media/ Basic media

Basal media are basically simple media that supports most non-fastidious bacteria. Peptone-water,nutrient broth,and nutrient agar(NA)are considered as basal medium. These media are generally used for the primary isolation of microorganisms.

Enriched medium (Added growth factors)

Blood agar addition of extra nutrients in the form of blood, serum, egg yolk, etc, to basal medium makes enriched media. *Enriched media are used to grow nutritionally exacting (fastidious) bacteria.* Blood agar, chocolate agar, Loeffler's serum slope, etc are few of the enriched media. Blood agar is prepared by adding 5-10% (by volume) blood to a blood agar base. **Chocolate agar** is also known as heated blood agar or lysed **blood agar.**

Selective and enrichment media

These media are designed to inhibit unwanted commensal or contaminating bacteria and help to recover pathogens from a mixture of bacteria. While selective media are agar-based, enrichment media are liquid in consistency. Both these media serve the same purpose. Any agar media can be made selective by the addition of certain inhibitory agents that don't affect the pathogen of interest. Various approaches to making a medium selective include addition of antibiotics, dycs, chemicals, alteration of pH, or a combination of these.

a. Selective medium

Principle: Differential growth suppression Selective medium is designed to suppress growth of some microorganisms while allowing the growth of others. Selective medium is agar-based (solid) medium so that individual colonies may be isolated.

Examples of selective media include

Thayer Martin Agar used to recover *Neisseria gonorrhoeae* contains antibiotics; vancomycin, colistin and nystatin.

Mannitol Salt Agar and Salt Milk Agar used to recover S.aureus contains 10% NaCl.

Potassium tellurite medium used to recover *C.diphtheriae* contains 0.04% potassium **MacConkey's Agar** used for **Enterobacteriaceae** members contains bile salt that inhibits most gram positive bacteria.

Pseudosol Agar (Cetrimide Agar) used to recover *P. aeruginosa* contains cetrimide (antiseptic agent).

Crystal Violet Blood Agar used to recover *S. pyogenes* contains 0.0002% crystal violet.

Lowenstein Jensen Medium used to recover *M.tuberculosis* is made selective by incorporating malachite green.

Wilson and Blair's Agar for recovering *S. typhi* is rendered selective by the addition of dye brilliant green.

Selective media such as **TCBS Agar** used for isolating *V. cholerae* from faecal specimens have elevated pH (8.5-8.6), which inhibits most other bacteria.

b. Enrichment culture medium

Enrichment medium is used to increase the relative concentration of certain microorganisms in the culture prior to plating on solid selective medium. Unlike selective media, enrichment culture is typically used as a broth medium. Enrichment media are liquid media that also serves to inhibit commensals in the clinical specimen. **Selenite F broth**, tetrathionate broth, and **alkaline peptone water (APW)** are used to recover pathogens from faecal specimens.

Differential/ indicator medium: differential appearance:

Certain media are designed in such a way that different bacteria can be recognized on the basis of their colony colour. Various approaches include incorporation of dyes, metabolic substrates, etc, so that those bacteria that utilize them appear as differently coloured colonies. Such media are called differential media or indicator media. Differential media allow the growth of more than one microorganism of interest but with morphologically distinguishable colonies.

Examples of differential media include

Mannitol salts agar (mannitol fermentation = yellow)

Blood agar (various kinds of hemolysis i.e. α, β and γ hemolysis)

Mac Conkey agar (lactose fermenters, pink colonies whereas non- lactose fermenter produces pale or colourless colonies.

TCBS (*Vibrio cholera* produces yellow colonies due to fermentation of sucrose)

Transport media

Clinical specimens must be transported to the laboratory immediately after collection to prevent overgrowth of contaminating organisms or commensals. This can be achieved by using transport media. Such media prevent drying (desiccation) of a specimen, maintain the pathogen to commensal ratio, and inhibit the overgrowth of unwanted bacteria. Some of these media (Stuart's & Amie's) are semi-solid in consistency. Addition of charcoal serves to neutralize inhibitory factors.

Cary Blair transport medium and Venkatraman Ramakrishnan (VR) medium are used to transport faeces from suspected cholera patients.

Sach's buffered glycerol saline is used to transport faeces from patients suspected to be suffering from bacillary dysentery.

Pike's medium is used to transport streptococci from throat specimens.

Anaerobic media

Anaerobic bacteria need special media for growth because they need low oxygen content, reduced oxidation-reduction potential and extra nutrients.

Media for anaerobes may have to be supplemented with nutrients like hemin and vitamin K. Such media may also have to be reduced by physical or chemical means. Boiling the medium serves to expel any dissolved oxygen. Addition of 1% glucose, 0.1% thioglycollate, 0.1% ascorbic acid, 0.05% cysteine, or red-hot iron filings can render a medium reduced. Before using the medium must be boiled in a water bath to expel any dissolved oxygen and then sealed with sterile liquid paraffin.

Robertson Cooked Meat (RCM) medium that is commonly used to grow *Clostridium* spps contains a 2.5 cm column of bullock heart meat and 15 ml of nutrient broth. **Thioglycollate** broth contains sodium thioglycollate, glucose, cystine, yeast extract and casein hydrolysate.

Methylene blue or resazurin is an oxidation-reduction potential indicator that is incorporated in the medium. Under reduced condition, methylene blue is colourless.

Assay media

These media are used for the assay of vitamins, amino acids, and antibiotics. E.g. antibiotic assay media are used for determining antibiotic potency by the microbiological assay technique.

Other types of medium include;

Media for enumeration of bacteria,

Media for characterization of bacteria,

Maintenance media etc.

Mueller-Hinton agar is a microbiological growth medium that is commonly used for antibiotic susceptibility testing. Originally formulated for isolation of *Neisseria* species.

It is also used to isolate and maintain *Neisseria* and *Moraxella* species.

Growth and Multiplication of Bacteria

Bacteria divide by binary fission. When a bacterial cell reaches a certain size, it divides to form two daughter cells. Nuclear division is followed by cell division. The interval of time between two cell divisions, or the time required for a bacterium to give rise to two daughter cells under optimum conditions, is called the generation time or the population doubling time. In Escherichia coli and many other medically important bacteria, the generation time is about 20 minutes. Some bacteria are slow-growing. The generation time in tubercle bacilli is about 20 hours. In leprae bacilli, it is as long as about 20 days. When bacteria are grown in a vessel of liquid medium, multiplication is arrested after a few cell divisions due to depletion of nutrients or accumulation of toxic products. This is a batch culture. By the use of special devices for replenishing nutrients and removing bacterial cells (chemostat or turbidostat), it is possible to maintain a continuous culture of bacteria for industrial or research purposes. When bacteria multiply in host tissues, the situation may be intermediate between a batch culture and a continuous culture. The source of nutrients may be inexhaustible but the bacteria have to fight the defence mechanisms of the host.

Bacteria growing on solid media (for example blood agar, MacConkey agar) form colonies. Each colony represents a cluster of cells derived from a parent cell. In liquid media, growth is diffuse. Bacterial growth may be considered at two levels: increase in the size of the bacterial cell and increase in the number of cells.

Growth in numbers can be studied by bacterial counts. Two types of bacterial counts can be made: total count and viable count. The total count gives the total number of cells in the sample, irrespective of whether they are living or not. It can be done by various methods, for example direct counting under the microscope using counting chambers. The viable count measures the number of living cells, that is, cells capable of multiplication. Viable counts are obtained by dilution or plating methods. In the dilution method, the suspension, whose cell count is to be determined, is serially diluted. The dilutions are made to the point beyond which unit quantities do not yield growth when inoculated into suitable liquid media. Each dilution is inoculated into the respective tubes containing liquid media. The viable count is statistically evaluated from the number of tubes showing growth. This method is not accurate but is used for the estimation of "presumptive coliform count" in drinking water. The presumptive coliform count is a method of estimating the level of pollution of drinking water. In the plating method, appropriate dilutions are inoculated on solid media, either on the surface of plates or as pour plates. The number of colonies that develop after incubation gives an estimate of the viable count. The method commonly employed is that described by Miles and Misra (1938) in which serial dilutions are dropped on the surface of dried plates and colony counts obtained.

Bacterial growth curve

When a bacterium is seeded into a suitable liquid medium and incubated, its growth follows a definite course. If bacterial counts are made at intervals after inoculation and plotted in relation to time, a growth curve is obtained.

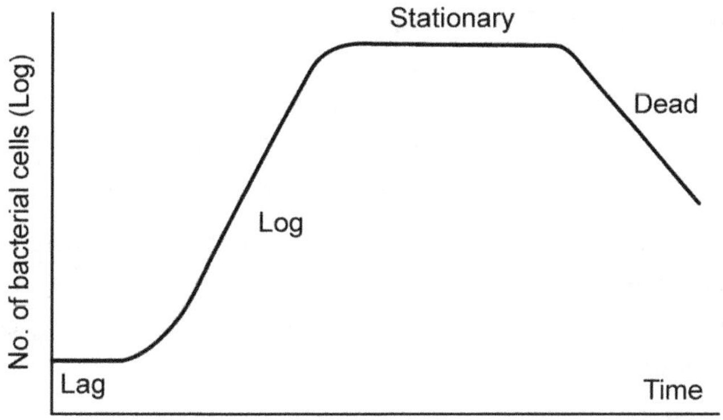

Fig 1.4. Bacterial growth curve.

The curve shows the following phases:

Lag phase: Immediately following the seeding of a culture medium, there is no appreciable increase in number, though there may be an increase in the size of the cells. This initial period is the time required for adaptation to the new environment. The necessary enzymes and metabolic intermediates are built up in adequate quantities for multiplication to proceed. The maximum cell size is obtained towards the end of lag phase. The duration of the lag phase varies with the species, size of the inoculum, nature of the culture medium and environmental factors such as temperature.

Log (logarithmic) or exponential phase: Following the lag phase, the cells start dividing and their numbers increase exponentially or by geometric progression with time. If the logarithm of the viable count is plotted against time, a straight line will be obtained. In this phase, cells are smaller and stain uniformly.

Stationary phase: After a varying period of exponential growth, cell division stops due to depletion of nutrients and accumulation of toxic products. The number of new cells formed is just enough to replace the number of cells that die. Equilibrium exists between the dying cells and the newly formed cells. So, the viable count remains stationary. In this phase, cells are frequently gram variable and show irregular staining. Sporulation occurs at this stage.

Phase of decline: This is the phase when the population decreases due to cell death. Besides nutritional exhaustion and toxic accumulation, cell death may also be caused by autolytic enzymes.

Isolation and preservation methods for pure cultures

Culture: Act of cultivating microorganisms or the microorganisms that are cultivated. Mixed culture has more than one microorganism.

Pure culture: containing a single species of organism.

A pure culture is usually derived from a mixed culture (one containing many species) by transferring a small sample into new, sterile growth medium in such a manner as to disperse the individual cells across the medium surface or by thinning the sample many times before inoculating the new medium.

Pure cultures are important in microbiology for the following reasons-

- Once purified, the isolated species can then be cultivated with the knowledge that only the desired microorganism is being grown.
- A pure culture can be correctly identified for accurate studying and testing, and diagnosis in a clinical environment.
- Testing/experimenting with a pure culture ensures that the same results can be achieved regardless of how many times the test is repeated.
- Pure culture spontaneous mutation rate is low
- Pure culture clone is 99.999% identical.

Common isolation techniques

Streak plate method, pour plate method, Spread plate method & Roll tube method.

Special methods of Isolation of Pure Culture

→ **Single cell isolation methods**
  → **Capillary pipette method**
  → **Micromanipulator method**

→ **Enrichment culture methods**

Streak plate method

Streaking is the process of spreading the needle on the surface of the media. Sterilize the inoculating needle by flame to make red hot and allow it to cool for 30seconds.

The sample is streaked in such a way to provide series of dilution. The purpose is to thin out inoculum to get separate colonies. Culturing can be done by streaking well isolated colonies from streak plate to new plate.

Pour plate method

The bacterial culture and liquid agar medium are mixed together. After mixing the medium, the medium containing the culture poured into sterilized Petri dishes (Petri plates), allowed solidifying and then incubated. After incubation colonies appear on the surface.

Demerits

1. Microorganism trapped beneath the surface of medium hence surface as well as subsurface colonies are developed which makes the difficulties in counting the bacterial colony.
2. Tedious and time-consuming method, microbes are subjected to heat shock because liquid medium maintained at 45°C.
3. Unsuitable-Psychrophile.

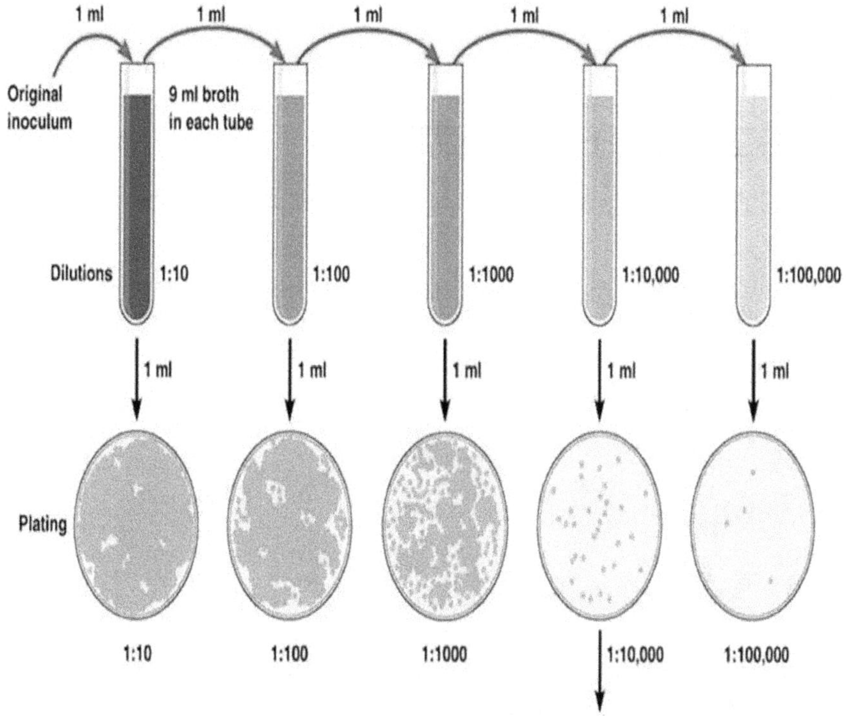

Calculation: Number of colonies on plate × reciprocal of dilution of sample = number of bacteria/ml
(For example, if 32 colonies are on a plate of 1/10,000 dilution, then the count is 32 × 10,000 = 320,000 bacteria/ml in sample.)

Spread plate method

This is the best method to isolate the pure colonies.

In this technique, the culture is not mixed with the normal saline and serially diluted agar medium. Instead, it is mixed with 0.1ml of sample taken from diluted mixture, which is placed on the surface of the agar plate and spread evenly over the surface by using L shaped glass rod called spreader.

Incubate the plates, after incubation, colonies are observed on the agar surface.

Merits/Advantages

It is a simple method. In this method only, surface colonies are formed. Micro-organisms are not exposed to higher temperature.

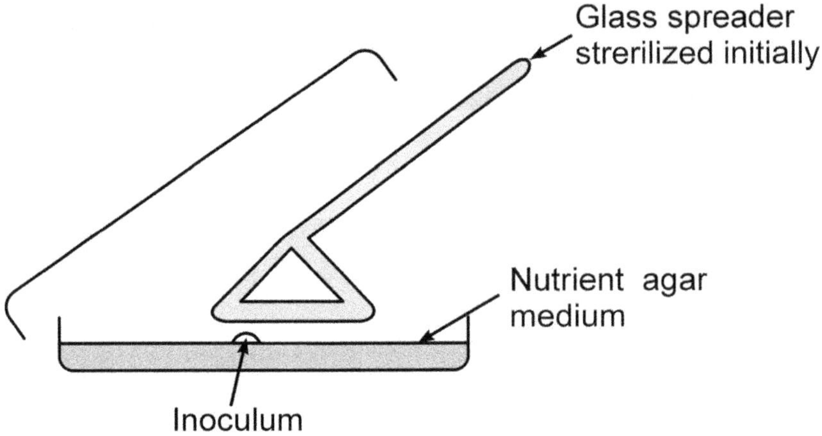

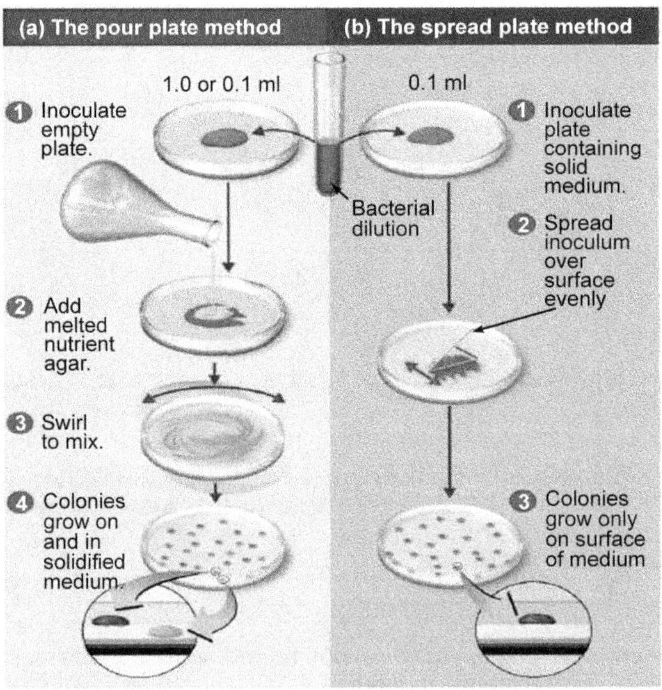

Pour plate method

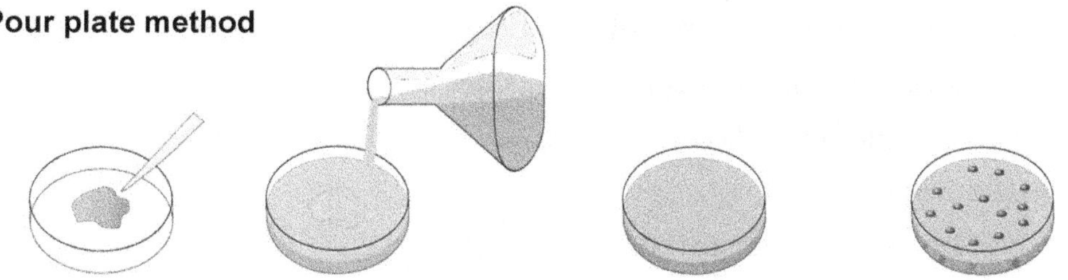

Spread plate method

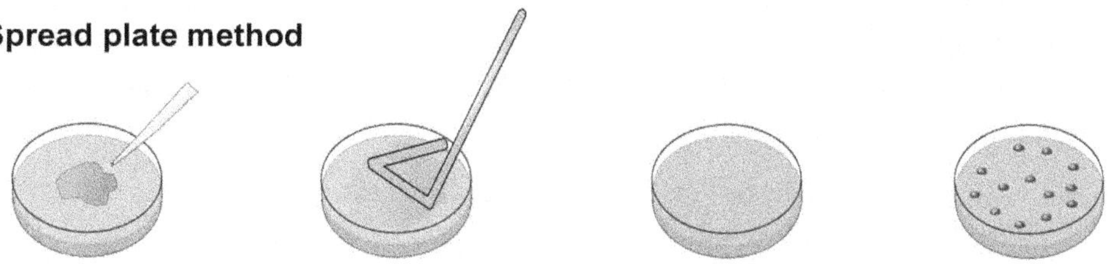

Roll tube method

A roll-tube method was developed in which agar medium was distributed as a thin layer over the internal surface of test tubes charged with an anaerobic atmosphere for the isolation of obligately anaerobic bacteria of the rumen. In the roll-tube method, exposure of bacteria and culture medium to air is avoided by displacing the air in the culture vessel with an oxygen-free gas, such as carbon dioxide, hydrogen, nitrogen, or mixtures of these gases. Carbon dioxide is the gas of choice because it is heavier than air, relatively cheap, and valuable in buffering. Vessels are stoppered under conditions preventing access of air. The cultures require no special incubators and can be removed and examined with no anaerobic precautions if kept stoppered. If opened, anaerobiosis can be continuously maintained during necessary manipulations, and the culture again closed without exposure to oxygen.

Micromanipulator method

Micromanipulators have been built, which permit one to pick out a single cell from a mixed culture. This instrument is used in conjunction with a microscope to pick a single cell (particularly bacterial cell) from a hanging drop preparation.

the single cell of microbe sucked into micropipette and transferred to large amount of sterile medium.

Advantages of micromanipulator method

The advantages of this method are that one can be reasonably sure from a single cell and one can obtain strains within the species.

Disadvantages

The disadvantages are that the equipment is expensive, its manipulation is very tedious, and it requires a skilled person.

Preservation of Pure Culture

To maintain pure culture for extended periods in viable condition without any genetic change is referred as Preservation. During preservation most important factor is to stop microbial growth or at least lower the growth rate.

Aim of Preservation

To maintain isolated pure culture for extended periods in a viable condition. To avoid contamination and to restrict Genetic Mutation.

Why to Preserve Bacteria

- In nature there are only 1% bacteria which is pathogenic and harmful to Animalia and Plantae.
- 99% of bacterial populations are of economic importance for human beings and plants.
- In soil for nutrient uptake in food industry, in sewage treatment, in medical industry.

So, the preservation of bacteria is one of the most profitable practices economically as well as environmentally. For Academic purpose, Research Purpose, Biotechnology field and in Fermentation Industry.

Preservation methods of Bacteria

1. Periodic transfer to fresh medium
2. Storage at low temperature
3. Storage in sterile soil
4. Preservation by overlaying culture with mineral oil
5. Lyophilization or freeze drying

Periodic transfer to fresh medium

Strains can be maintained by periodically preparina fresh culture from the previous stock culture. The culture medium, the storage temperature, and the time transfers are made vary with the species.

The temperature and the type of medium chosen should support a slow rather than a rapid rate of growth so that the time interval between transfers can be as long as possible. Many of the more common heterotrophs remain viable for several weeks or months on a medium like Nutrient Agar. The transfer method has the disadvantage of failing to prevent changes in the characteristics of a strain due to the development of variants and mutants.

Storage at Low Temperature

By Refrigeration & Cryopreservation Pure cultures can be successfully stored at 0-4°C either in refrigerators or in cold-rooms.

This method is applied for short duration (2-3 weeks for bacteria and 3-4 months for fungi) because the metabolic activities of the microorganisms are greatly slowed down but not stopped.

Thus, their growth continue slowly, nutrients are utilized and waste products released in medium.

This results in finally the death of the micro-organism.

Cryopreservation

Cryopreservation (i.e., freezing in liquid nitrogen at -196°C or in the gas phase above the liquid nitrogen at -150°C) helps survival of pure cultures for long storage times.

In this method, the microorganisms of culture are rapidly frozen in liquid nitrogen at - 196°C in the presence of stabilizing agents such as glycerol or Dimethyl Sulfoxide (DMSO) that prevent the cell damage due to formation of ice crystals and promote cell survival.

This liquid nitrogen method has been successful with many species that cannot be preserved by lyophilization and most species can remain viable under these conditions for 10 to 30 years without undergoing change in their characteristics, however this method is expensive.

Storage in sterile soil

Storing organisms in soil fall into two groups

Sterile soil infested with small amount of inoculum, immediately dried and stored in refrigerator. Soil infested with the organism, then incubated allowing

The organism to grow thus, the mycelium and propagative unit of second generation are preserved. The soil preservation method is useful for fungi, and by this method actinomycetes are maintained in soil for 4 to 5 years, and there are several bacterial spp which are also maintained in soil for several years.

Merits

We can remove some of the growth under the oil with a transfer needle, inoculate afresh medium, and still preserve the original culture. The simplicity of the method makes it attractive, but changes in the characteristics of a strain can still occur.

Paraffin Method/Preservation by Overlaying Cultures with Mineral Oil

- Simple, most economical method. Agar slants are inoculated & incubated.
- Then, covered with sterile mineral oil to a depth of 1cm above the tip of slant surface.
- Transfers are made by removing a loop full of growth touching the tip to the glass surface to drain off excess il-inoculating a fresh medium-preserving the initial stock culture.
- Functions-provinding an aerobic condition, prevents the dehydration of the medium and decreases the metabolic rate of the organisms.

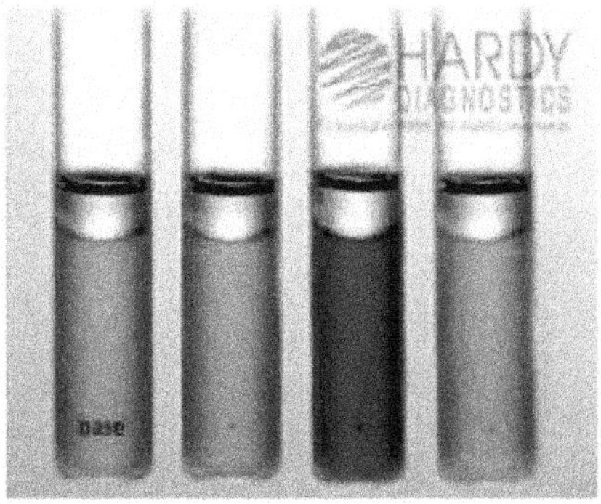

Lyophilization or freeze drying

Freeze drying is a stabilizing process in which a substance is first frozen and then the quantity of the solvent is reduced, first by sublimation (primary drying stage) and then desorption (secondary drying stage).

Better preservation occurs with freeze-drying than with other methods because freeze-drying reduces the risk of intracellular ice crystallization that compromises viability, removal of water from specimen effectively prevents this damage. Lyophilisation is greatest with gram-positive bacteria (spore formers) and decrease with gram -negative bacteria but viability can be maintained as long as 30 years.

Large numbers of vials of dried microorganisms can be stored with limited space, and organisms can be easily transported long distances at room temperature. The process combines freezing and dehydration- Organisms are initially frozen and then dried by lowering the atmospheric pressure with a vacuum apparatus. Specimens can be connected individually to the condenser (manifold method) or can be placed (in a chamber) where they are dehydrated in one larger airspace.

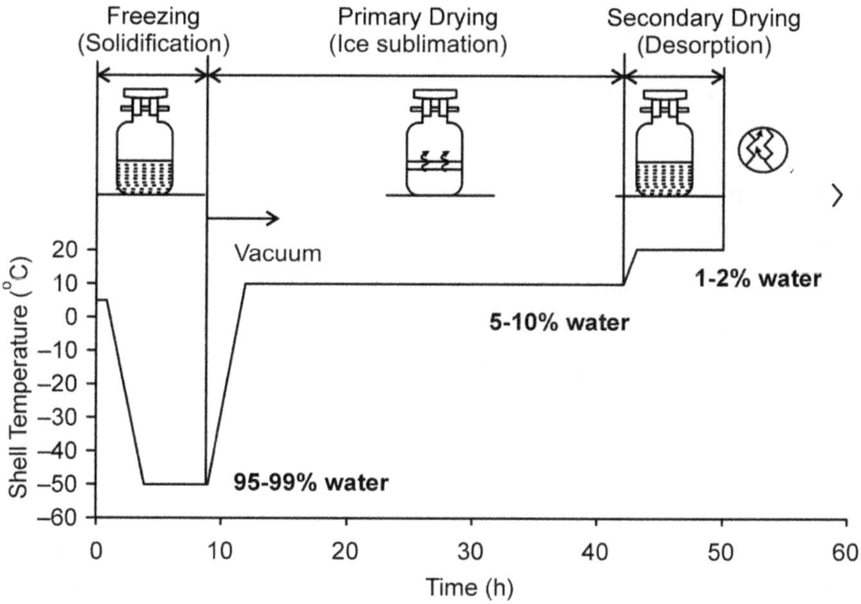

Storage Vials

Glass vials are used for all freeze-dried specimens. When freeze-drying is performed in a chamber, double glass vials are used.

Chamber method: an outer soft glass for protection and preservation of the dehydrated specimen. Silica gel granulesare placed in the bottom vial before the inner vial is inserted and cushioned with cotton.

Manifold method - a single glass vial is used. storage vial must be sealed to maintain the vacuum and the dry atmospheric condition.

Cryoprotective Agents Most commonly used agent is Skim milk for chamber lyophilisation.

Advantages: Removal of water at low temperature, Thermolabile materials can be dried, Sterility can be maintained, Reconstitution is easy.

Disadvantages

Many biological molecules are damaged by the stress associated with freezing, freeze- drying, or both. E.g. the process of drying causes extensive damage to moulds, protozoa, and most viruses, Hence, these microorganisms cannot be stored by this method. The product is prone to oxidation, due to high porosity and large surface area. Therefore, the product should be packed in vacuum or using inert gas.

Anaerobic bacteria culture

An anaerobic bacteria culture is a method used to grow anaerobes from a clinical specimen. Obligate anaerobes are bacteria that can live only in the absence of oxygen. Obligate anaerobes are destroyed when exposed to the atmosphere for as briefly as 10 minutes. Some anaerobes are tolerant to small amounts of oxygen. Facultative anaerobes are those organisms that will grow with or without oxygen. The methods of obtaining specimens for anaerobic culture and the culturing procedure are performed to ensure that the organisms are protected from oxygen.

Cultivation of Anaerobic Bacteria

Main Principle is to reduce the O_2 content of culture medium and remove any oxygen already present inside the system or in the medium.

Oxygen is ubiquitous in the air so special methods are needed to culture anaerobic microorganisms. A number of procedures are available for reducing the O2 content of cultures; some simple but suitable mainly for less sensitive organisms, others more complex but necessary for growth of strict anaerobes.

Bottles or tubes filled completely to the top with culture medium and provided with tightly fitting stopper. Suitable for organisms not too sensitive to small amounts of oxygen.

Addition of a reducing agent that reacts with oxygen and reduces it to water e.g., Thioglycolate in thioglycolate broth. After thioglycolate reacts with oxygen throughout the tube, oxygen can penetrate only near the top of the tube where the medium contacts air.

Obligate aerobes grow only at the top of such tubes. Facultative organisms grow throughout the tube but best near the top. Microaerophiles grow near the top but not right at the top. Anaerobes grow only near the bottom of the tube, where oxygen cannot penetrate. redox indicator dye called resazurin is added to the medium because the dye changes colour in the presence of oxygen and thereby indicates the degree of penetration of oxygen into the medium.

Strict anaerobes, such as methanogenic bacteria can be killed by even a brief exposure to O_2. In these cases, a culture medium is first boiled to render it oxygen free, and then a reducing agent such as H_2S is added and the mixture is sealed under an oxygen- free gas. All manipulations are carried out under a tiny jet of oxygen free hydrogen or nitrogen gas that is directed into the culture vessel when it is open, thus driving out any O_2 that might enter. For extensive research on anaerobes, special boxes fitted with gloves, called anaerobic glove boxes, permit work with open cultures in completely anoxic atmospheres.

Stringent anaerobes can be grown only by taking special precautions to exclude all atmospheric oxygen from the medium. Such an environment can be established by using one of the following methods:

Pre-reduced media

During preparation, the culture medium is boiled for several minutes to drive off most of the dissolved oxygen. A reducing agent e.g., cysteine, is added to further lower the oxygen content. Oxygen free N2 is bubbled through the medium to keep it anaerobic. The medium is then dispensed into tubes which are being flushed with oxygen – free nitrogen, stoppered tightly, and sterilized by autoclaving. Such tubes are continuously flushed with oxygen free CO2 by means of a cannula, restoppered, and incubatcd.

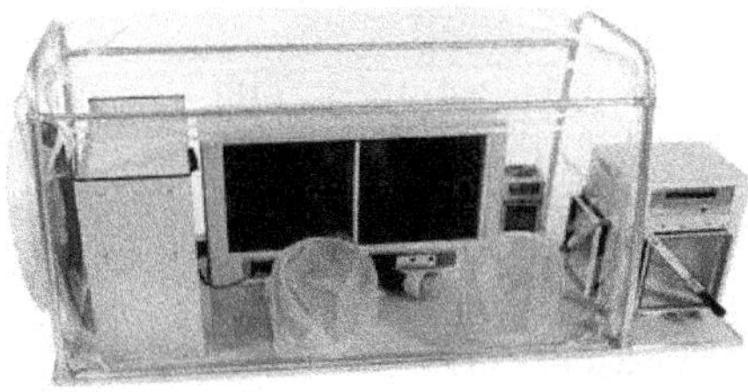

Fig 1.5. Anaerobic Chambers.

1. Anaerobic Chamber

This refers to a plastic anaerobic glove box that contains an atmosphere of H_2, CO_2, and N_2. Culture media are placed within the chamber by means of an air lock which can be evacuated and refilled with N_2. Any oxygen in the media is slowly removed by reaction with hydrogen, forming water; this reaction is aided by a palladium catalyst. After being rendered oxygen free, the media are inoculated within the chamber (by means of the glove ports) and incubated (also within the chamber).

2. Anaerobic Jar

GasPak systemAnaerobic jar is a heavy- walled jar with a gas tight seal within which tubes, plates, or other containers to be incubated are placed along with H_2 and CO_2 generating system (**GasPak system**). After the jar is sealed oxygen present in the atmosphere inside jar and dissolved in the culture medium, is gradually used up through reaction with the hydrogen in the presence of catalyst. The air in the jar is replaced with a mixture of H_2 and CO_2, thus leading to anoxic conditions.

Counting of microorganisms:

Counting of microorganisms can be done by different methods. In most cases the sample to be counted is first diluted to avoid overwhelming the whole counting procedure. However, in some cases, the sample may be too dilute to give the required minimum count to be able to estimate the microbial population of that sample. In such cases, concentration of the sample is carried out.

Counting can be done by use of a slide and a cover slip. A drop of the diluted sample is put on the slide with a suitable agent for proper visualization of the sample. It is then covered with a cover slip and put under a microscope and observed at a suitable magnification. The centre area can be dimensioned with etched grids. The number of microbes in the grids is multiplied by the dilution factor to get the number in the original sample.

The Petri dish count is where the sample is diluted to a point where the colonies will be statistically significant to be counted but not so many to overgrow each other. This method takes time for the individual cells to grow into colonies. The colonies counted are multiplied by the dilution factor to get the number in the original sample. The results here are expressed in colony forming units per milli liter i.e. CFU/ML. The time taken for the cells to grow into individual colonies is called the incubation period.

Total count:

Total count is also termed as standard plate count or colony count. It gives the total number of microbes both viable and non-viable. All cells are counted. These include bacteria, yeasts and moulds. It is usually done by pour plate method. Total count generally requires employment of a microscope.

For instance, when determining total microbial count in water by pour plate, a known volume of water is mixed with molten yeast-malt extract agar and given time to solidify. This is done on several plates. One set of plates are incubated at 37°C for about 24 hours and the other set of plates are incubated at 20-22°C for 3 days. Most bacteria capable of growth in water do so well at 22°C than at higher temperatures. While the microbes that grow well at 37°C will not grow very well in water. This means that the two types of microorganisms need to be counted differently since they differ in their growth pattern. In this case, carrying out of total count on water is beneficial in several ways.

It helps to evaluate the efficiency of certain water treatment processes like coagulation, flocculation and disinfection. It also gives an indication of the level of cleanliness of the water distribution system. It can also be used it determine the suitability of water supply to firms where food and drinks are prepared on large scale.

Total count is achieved either by use of direct or indirect counts. One method of direct count is the use of a haemocytometer. A haemocytometer is a specialized microscope slide important in cell counting. The central part of this slide has etched grids with precisely spaced lines to enable accurate counting. In order to get an accurate count in this method, the cell number should range between 40 to 70 cells in a one mm square. If this requirement is not met, necessary adjustments by either dilution or concentration are done as necessary.

In indirect counts, one method is by use of a colorimeter. As the microorganisms grow with time, they make the agar more and more turbid. This turbidity can be measured by use of a colorimeter where optical density is measured. The greater the optical density the greater the number of microbes.

There is also a measure of dry weight. This method involves centrifugation followed by weighing to get the dry weight. The limitation of this method is that cells are destroyed.

The other indirect count method involves the use of a coulter counter. A coulter counter is a probe which measures variation in conductivity of a solution as a bacteria passes through a narrow gap.

The advantage of direct and indirect counts is that the process can be automated but the disadvantage is that they cannot differentiate dead cells from living ones.

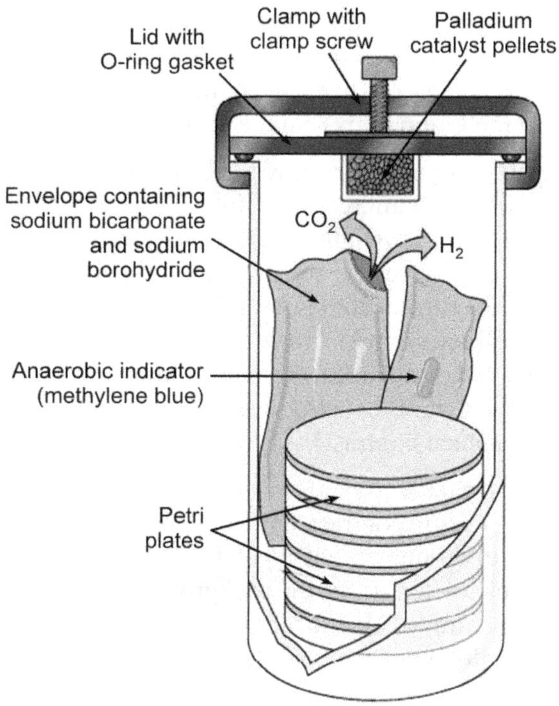

Viable count:

Viable count involves counting of colonies produced by only viable cells under favourable growth conditions. This can be accomplished by techniques like pour plating, spread plating and most probable number with an assumption that each and every viable cell gives rise to a pure colony.

In pour plating, the liquid media and the diluted sample are poured together in Petri dishes while still in liquid form and left to solidify. After solidifying, the Petri dishes are incubated at appropriate temperature for the required period of time during which the growth is realized. The plates are then removed and distinct colonies counted and expressed in colony forming units per ml.

Phase-Contrast Microscopy

Phase-contrast microscopy visualizes differences in the refractive indexes of different parts of a specimen relative to unaltered light.

Phase-contrast microscopy is a method of manipulating light paths through the use of strategically placed rings in order to illuminate transparent objects. Dutch physicist Fritz Zernike developed the technique in the 1930s; for his efforts he was awarded the Nobel Prize in 1953. In phase-contrast microscopy, parallel beams of light are passed through objects of different densities. The microscope contains special condensers that throw light "out of phase" causing it to pass through the object at different speeds. Internal details and organelles of live, unstained organisms (e.g. mitochondria, lysosomes, and the Golgi body) can be seen clearly with this microscope.

A phase ring in condenser allows a cylinder of light to pass through it while still in phase. Unaltered light hits the phase ring in the lens and is excluded. Light that is slightly altered by passing through a different refractive index is allowed to pass through. Light passing through cellular structures, such as chromosomes or mitochondria is retarded because they have a higher refractive index than the surrounding medium. Elements of lower refractive index advance the wave. Much of the background light is removed and light that constructively or destructively interfered is let through with enhanced contrast.

Phase-contrast microscopy allows the visualization of living cells in their natural state with high contrast and high resolution. This tool works best with a thin specimen and is not ideal for a thick specimen. Phase-contrast images have a characteristic grey background with light and dark features found across the sample. One disadvantage of phase-contrast microscopy is halo formation called halo-light ring.

Electron Microscopy

Electron microscopy uses magnetic coils to direct a beam of electrons from a tungsten filament through a specimen and onto a monitor.

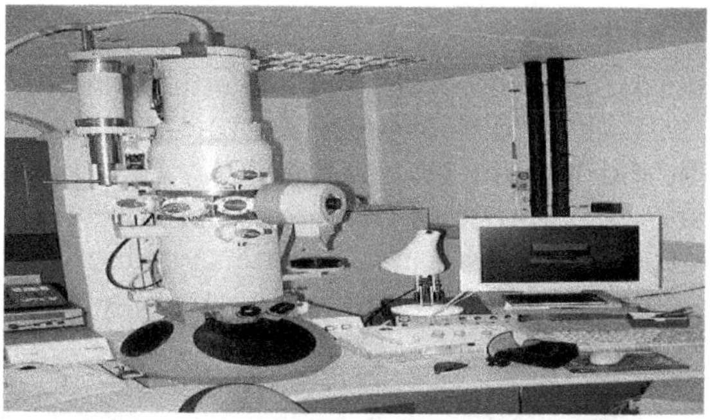

Fig 1.6. Electron Microscope a Modern Electron Microscope.

Electron microscopy uses a beam of electrons as an energy source. An electron beam has an exceptionally short wavelength and can hit most objects in its path, increasing the resolution of the final image captured. The electron beam is designed to travel in a vacuum to limit interference by air molecules. Magnets are used to focus the electrons on the object viewed.

There are two types of electron microscopes. The more traditional form is the transmission electron microscope (TEM). To use this instrument, ultra-thin slices of microorganisms or viruses are placed on a wire grid and then stained with gold or palladium before viewing, to create contrast. The densely coated parts of the specimen deflect the electron beam and both dark and light areas show up on the image. TEM can project images in a much higher resolution—up to the atomic level of thinner objects.

The second and most contemporary form is the scanning electron microscope (SEM). It allows the visualization of microorganisms in three dimensions as the electrons are reflected when passed over the specimen. The same gold or palladium staining is employed.

Electron microscopy has multiple applications. It is ideal to:

- explore the in vivo molecular mechanisms of disease;
- visualize the three-dimensional architecture of tissues and cells;
- determine the conformation of flexible protein structures and complexes;
- observe individual viruses and macromolecular complexes in their natural context.

Sample preparation can be critical to generate a successful image because the choice of reagents and methods used to process a sample largely depends on the nature of the sample and the analysis required.

Dark-Field Microscopy

Dark-field microscopes show a light silhouette of an organism against a dark background. In dark-field microscopy, the light reaches the specimen from an angle with the help of an opaque disk. The specimen appears lit up against a dark back ground. Dark-field microscopy is most useful for extremely small living organisms that are invisible in the light microscope Dark-field microscopes show a light silhouette of an organism against a dark background. Radiance Against a Dark Background

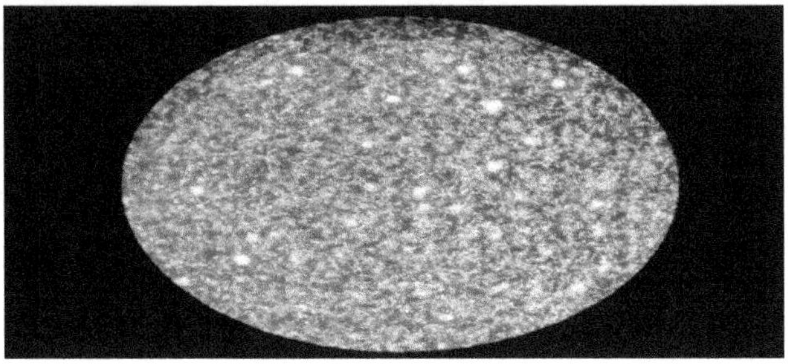

Fig 1.7. Visualization of live bacteria: Spirochetes bacteria observed under dark field microscopy.

Dark-field microscopy is ideally used to illuminate unstained samples causing them to appear brightly lit against a dark background. This type of microscope contains a special condenser that scatters light and causes it to reflect off the specimen at an angle. Rather than illuminating the sample with a filled cone of light, the condenser is designed to form a hollow cone of light. The light at the apex of the cone is focused at the plane of the specimen; as this light moves past the specimen plane it spreads again into a hollow cone. The objective lens sits in the dark hollow of this cone; although the light travels around and past the objective lens, no rays enter it.

The entire field appears dark when there is no sample on the microscope stage; thus the name dark-field microscopy. When a sample is on the stage, the light at the apex of the cone strikes it. The rays scattered by the sample and captured in the objective lens thus make the image.

Samples observed under dark-field microscopy should be carefully prepared since dust and other particles also scatter the light and are easily detected. Glass slides need to be thoroughly cleaned of extraneous dust and dirt. It may be necessary to filter sample media (agar, water, saline) to exclude confusing contaminants. Sample materials need to be spread thinly; too much material on the slide creates many overlapping layers and edges, making it difficult to interpret structures.

Dark-field microscopy has many applications in microbiology. It allows the visualization of live bacteria, and distinguishes some structure (rods, curved rods, spirals, or cocci) and movement.

UNIT - II

Staining & Sterilization

Identification of bacteria using staining techniques (simple, Gram's & Acid-fast staining) and biochemical tests (IMViC). Study of principle, procedure, merits, demerits and applications of physical, chemical gaseous, radiation and mechanical method of sterilization. Evaluation of the efficiency of sterilization methods. Equipment employed in large scale sterilization. Sterility indicators.

Introduction

Samples of blood, tissue, water, food and cosmetics are examined daily in laboratories throughout the world for checking the presence of contaminants and pathogenic microorganisms. Pharma industries and research institutes are constantly screening soil, water, marine samples to isolate new antibiotics, enzymes and vitamins producing microorganisms. Bergey's Manual of Systemic Bacteriology (BMSB) has been the official, Internationally accepted reference for bacterial classification.

Staining reactions

To study size, shape, arrangement and properties and different specific groups of microorganisms, Biological stains are used. Stains are organic compounds. Different types of staining techniques are used to study the morphological and structural properties of microorganisms.

Staining techniques

1. Simple staining
2. Negative staining
3. Gram staining
4. Acid-fast staining
5. Biological tests (Imvic test).

Simple Staining

Used only single stain Eg: Any one at a time- Methylene blue (2 - 3mins), Crystal violet (1-2mins), Carbol fuschin (15-30secs), Safranin (1mins), Malachite green(1-2mins), etc. Used to study Size, shape and bacterial cell arrangements. Basic stains with a positively charged chromogens (any substance that can become a pigment or colouring matter, as a substance in organic fluids that forms coloured compounds when oxidized, or a compound, not itself a dye, that can become a dye) are used. Used to elucidate the morphology and arrangement of bacterial cells.

Steps involved in simple staining

Select oil/grease free slide. Do it by washing with detergent and wiping the excess water and then dry the slide by passed through flame. These slide is allowed to air dry and smear of sample is applied. After air drying these slide is rapidly passed through a flame for three to four times for heat fixation. After heat fixation the slide is flooded with a particular stain and these stain is allowed to react for two-three minutes. Further the slide is washed under running distilled water. The slide is air dried and watched under oil immersion microscope.

Principle behind the simple staining

A stain has an ability to bind a cellular component. These abilities depend upon the charges present on cellular component and charges present on chromophore group of stain. Bacteria has large number of carboxyl group on its surface and these carboxyl group has negative charge. When these carboxyl group carry out ionization reaction it shows COO– and H+.

Acidic stains include eosin, acid fuchsin, rose bengal, and congo red. Basic stains include methylene blue, crystal violet, malachite green, basic fuchsin, carbolfuchsin, and safranin. Basic dyes are available as salts of acids Eg: Methylene blue chloride (MB.Cl , Malachite green chloride (MG.Cl) When these are ionised, MB.Cl Ionisation MB+ + Cl-. On addition to methylene blue for staining, exchange of MB+ with Na+ on the bacterial cell take place. Thus, when colouring agent forms ionic bond with cell or cell components, it results into the staining of cell. Concentration of MB is 0.5-2% in water.

Negative staining

Colouring the background of object, not stain but made visible against dark background. Bacteria are mixed with acidic stains such as Eosin or Nigrosine that provide a uniformly coloured background against which the unstained bacteria stand out in contrast. Useful to observed bacteria that are difficult to stain (Spirilli & spirochetes– Treponema pallidum, Borrelia burgdorferi, Leptospira). Acidic stains has negative charge; therefore, it doesn't combine with negatively charge on bacteria cell surface. Advantages over Simple: Natural size and shape of microorganism can be seen. Heat fixation is not required. Doesn't need physical and chemical treatment. It is possible to observe bacteria that are difficult to stain. The most commonly used negative staining reagents are uranyl acetate and uranyl formate.

Gram staining

Dr. HANS CHRISTIAN GRAM - Danish bacteriologist noted for his development of the Gram stain in 1884. It is used to differentiate bacterial species into two broad groups, Gram positive & Gram negative based on the physical property of their cell wall.

Gram staining is not only reveals the size and shape of bacteria but also used to differentiate bacteria into Gram positive and Gram negative cells. Hence, called differential staining. It is first and usually the only method employed for the diagnostic identification of bacteria in clinical specimens. Provides more information about the characteristics of the cell wall (thickness).

Thin smear of bacterial culture was made on clean glass slide. Then the slide air dried and heat fixed. Smear was covered with crystal violet for 30 seconds. The slide was washed with distilled water. Smear was covered with Grams iodine solution for 60 seconds. Slide was washed with 95% ethyl alcohol and then distilled water. Again the smear was covered with safranin for 30 seconds. Washed with distilled water and blot dried. Air dried and observed under microscope.

Principle: Violet dye and the iodine combine to form an insoluble, dark purple compound in the bacterial protoplasm and cell wall. This compound is dissociable in the decolourizer, which dissolves and removes its two components from the cell. But the removal is much slower from Gram-positive than from the Gram-negative bacteria, so that by correct timing the former stay dark purple whilst the latter become colourless. The difference between the two types of bacteria is that the Gram positive have thicker and denser peptidoglycan layers in their cell walls, which makes them less permeable to the stain than those of the Gram negative bacteria. The iodine has a critical role in enhancing this difference. It seems to bind temporarily to the peptidoglycan and make it even less permeable to the dye.

Acid fast staining

Another widely used differential staining procedure in bacteriology developed by Ehrlich in 1882. Also known as Ziehl–Neelsen staining. Some bacteria (specially M. Tuberculosis, Nocardia asteroides, Actinomycetes, and M. leprae) resist toward the gram staining or other staining due to high lipid content in the cell wall, hence they are called ACID FAST BACTERIA. Because of high lipid content, acid fast cell have low permeability to dyes and hence difficult to stain. 5% aqueous phenol and heat (physical intensifier) are used to enhance the penetration of primary stain (chemical intensifier). Classified into two group - A) **acid fast bacteria** B) **non-acid fast bacteria**. Acid-fast cells contain a large amount of lipids and waxes in their cell walls primarily mycolic acid.

Procedure: A clean sterile glass slide was taken. A thin uniform smear was prepared in the slide using an inoculation loop. The smear was allowed to air dry and then heat fixed. The smear was flooded with Ziehl-Neelsen Carbol Fuschin (ZNCF) and heated until steam arises. Preparation was allowed to stay for 5-7 min. The stain must not be allowed to evaporate or dry in the slide. Pour more carbol fuschin on slide if necessary. It is then washed under a low steam of running water. The smear was decolorized with 20% sulphuric acid OR 3% HCl + 95% ethanol. The slide is then washed again under running distilled water. Counter stain the smear with Methylene blue/Malachite green for the 2 min. Washed under running tap water. Slide was blot dried and examined under microscope.

IMViC test:

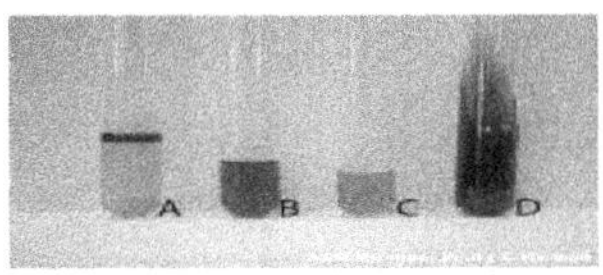

Fig.2.1 IMViC test for E Coli.

IMViC REACTIONS

IMViC reactions are a set of four useful reactions that are commonly employed in the identification of members of family entero bacteriaceae. The four reactions are: Indole test, Methyl Red test, Voges Proskauer test and Citrate utilization test. The letter "i" is only for rhyming purpose.

INDOLE TEST:

$$\text{Tryptophan} \xrightarrow[H_2O]{\text{tryptophanase}} \text{Indole} + \text{pyruvic acid} + NH_3$$

Principle: Some bacteria can produce indole from amino acid tryptophan using the enzyme typtophanase.

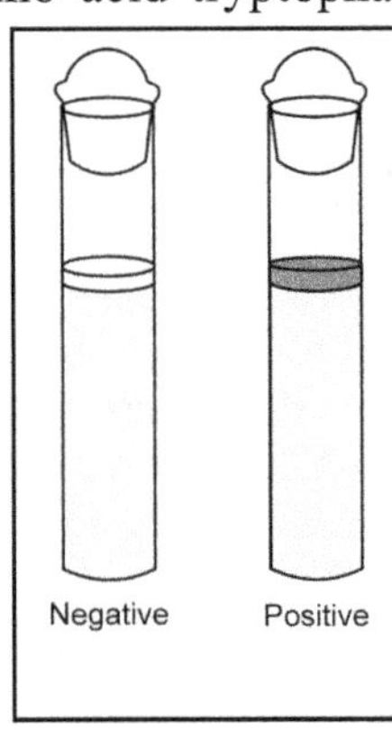

Production of indole is detected using Ehrlich's reagent or Kovac's reagent. Indole reacts with the aldehyde in the reagent to give a red color. An alcoholic layer concentrates the red color as a ring at the top.

Procedure: Bacterium to be tested is inoculated in peptone water, which contains amino acid tryptophan and incubated overnight at 37°C. Following incubation few drops of Kovac's reagent are added. Kovac's reagent consists of para-dimethyl amino benzaldehyde, isoamyl alcohol and Con. HCl. Ehrlich's reagent is more sensitive in detecting indole production in anerobes and non-fermenters. Formation of a red or pink coloured ring at the top is taken as positive.

Example: *Escherichia coli*: Positive; *Klebsiella pneumoniae*: Negative

METHYL RED (MR) TEST:

Principle: This is to detect the ability of an organism to produce and maintain stable acid end products from glucose fermentation. Some bacteria produce large amount of acids from glucose fermentation that they overcome the buffering action of the system. Methyl Red is a pH indicator, which remains red in color at a pH of 4.4 or less.

Procedure: the bacterium to be tested in inoculated into glucose phosphate broth, which contains glucose and a phosphate buffer and incubated at 37°C for 48 hours. Over the 48 hours the mixed-acid producing organism must produce sufficient acid to overcome the phosphate buffer and remain acid. The pH of the medium is tested by the addition of 5 drops of MR reagent. Development of red color is taken as positive. MR negative organism produce yellow color.

Example: *Eschericihia coli*: Positive and *Klebsiella pneumoniae*: Negative

VOGES PROSKAUER (VP) TEST

Principle: While MR test is useful in detecting mixed acid producers, VP test detects butylene glycol producers.

$$\text{Glucose} \longrightarrow \text{Acetoin}$$

$$\text{Acetoin} \xrightarrow[\text{atmospheric } O_2]{\text{KOH}} \text{Diacetyl} + H_2O$$

$$\text{Diacetyl} + \begin{array}{c}\text{guanidine}\\\text{component}\\\text{of peptone}\end{array} \xrightarrow{\text{alpha-naphthol}} \text{pink color}$$

Acetyl-methyl carbinol (acetoin) is an intermediate in the production of butylene glycol. In this test two reagents, 40% KOH and alpha-naphthol are added to test broth after incubation and exposed to atmospheric oxygen. If acetoin is present, it is oxidized in the presence of air and KOH to diacetyl. Diacetyl then reacts with guanidine components of peptone, in the presence of alpha- naphthol to produce red color. Role of alpha-naphthol is that of a catalyst and a color intensifier.

Procedure: Bacterium to be tested is inoculated into glucose phosphate broth and incubated for at least 48 hours. 0.6 ml of alpha-naphthol is added to the test broth and shaken. 0.2 ml of 40% KOH is added to the broth and shaken. The tube is allowed to stand for 15 minutes. Appearance of red color is taken as a positive test. The negative tubes must be held for one hour, since maximum color development occurs within one hour after addition of reagents.

Examples: *Escherichia coli*: Negative; and *Klebsiella pneumoniae*: Positive

CITRATE UTILIZATION TEST

$$\text{Citrate} \longrightarrow \text{Oxaloacetate} + \text{Acetate}$$

$$\text{Oxaloacetate} \longrightarrow \text{Pyruvate} + CO_2$$

$$CO_2 + Na + H_2O \longrightarrow Na_2CO_3$$

Principle: This test detects the ability of an organism to utilize citrate as the sole source of carbon and energy. Bacteria are inoculated on a medium containing sodium citrate and a pH indicator bromothymol blue. The medium also contains inorganic ammonium salts, which is utilized as sole source of nitrogen.

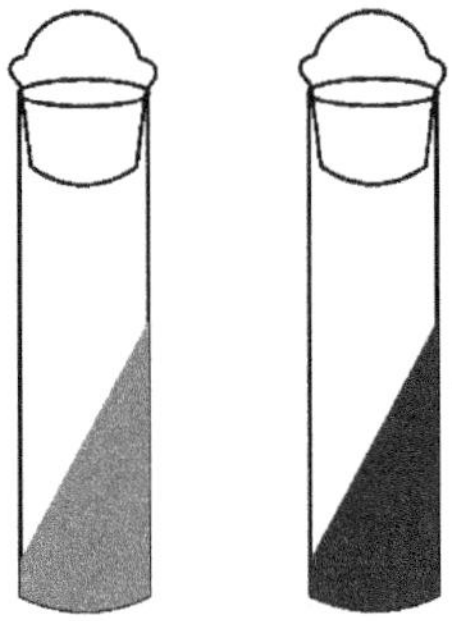

Negative Positive

Utilization of citrate involves the enzyme citritase, which breaks down citrate to oxaloacetate and acetate. Oxaloacetate is further broken down to pyruvate and CO_2. Production of Na_2CO_3 as well as NH_3 from utilization of sodium citrate and ammonium salt respectively result in alkaline pH. This results in change of medium's color from green to blue.

Procedure: Bacterial colonies are picked up from a straight wire and inoculated into slope of Simmon's citrate agar and incubated overnight at 37°C. If the organism has the ability to utilize citrate, the medium changes its color from green to blue.

Examples: *Escherichia coli*: Negative; *Klebsiella pneumoniae*: Positive

Bacterium	Indole	MR	VP	Citrate
E. coli	+	+	-	-
K. pneumoniae	-	-	+	+

WHAT IS STERILIZATION

Sterilization can be defined as any process that effectively kills or eliminates transmissible agents (such as fungi, bacteria, viruses and prions) from a surface, equipment, foods, medications, or biological culture medium.

The various methods of sterilization are:

1. **Physical Method**
   (a) Thermal methods (Dry and Moist heat)
   (b) Radiation method
   (c) Filtration method
2. **Chemical Method**
   (a) Gaseous method

Physical methods

1. **Heat sterilization:**

Heat sterilization is the most widely used and reliable method of sterilization, involving destruction of enzymes and other essential cell constituents. This method of sterilization can be applied only to the thermo stable products and moisture- sensitive materials.

(i) Dry Heat (160-1800°C) - Sterilization for thermostable products

(ii) Moist heat (121-1340 °C) - Sterilization is used for moisture- resistant materials.

The efficiency with which heat is able to inactivate microorganisms is dependent upon: The degree of heat, the exposure time and the presence of water.

The action of heat will be due to induction of lethal chemical events mediated through the action of water and oxygen.

In the presence of water much lower temperature time exposures are required to kill microbe than in the absence of water.

***Thermal methods include*:**

I Dry Heat Sterilization

Ex: 1. Incineration 2. Red heat 3. Flaming 4. Hot air oven

II Moist Heat Sterilization

Ex: 1. Dry saturated steam – Autoclaving 2. Boiling water/steam at atmospheric pressure 3. Hot water below boiling point.

Physical methods for Sterilization

Sunlight

The microbicidal activity of sunlight is mainly due to the presence of ultra violet rays in it. It is responsible for spontaneous sterilization in natural conditions. In tropical countries, the sunlight is more effective in killing germs due to combination of ultraviolet rays and heat. By killing bacteria suspended in water, sunlight provides natural method of disinfection of water bodies such as tanks and lakes.

Heat

Heat is considered to be most reliable method of sterilization of articles that can withstand heat. Heat acts by oxidative effects as well as denaturation and coagulation of proteins. Those articles that cannot withstand high temperatures can still be sterilized at lower temperature by prolonging the duration of exposure.

Factors affecting sterilization by heat

Nature of heat: Moist heat is more effective than dry heat.

Temperature and time: temperature and time are inversely proportional. As temperature increases the time taken decreases.

Number of microorganisms: More the number of microorganisms, higher the temperature or longer the duration required.

Nature of microorganism: Depends on species and strain of microorganism, sensitivity to heat may vary. Spores are highly resistant to heat.

Type of material: Articles that are heavily contaminated require higher temperature or prolonged exposure. Certain heat sensitive articles must be sterilized at lower temperature.

Presence of organic material: Organic materials such as protein, sugars, oils and fats increase the time required.

Action of heat

Dry heat acts by protein denaturation, oxidative damage and toxic effects of elevated levels of electrolytes.

The moist heat acts by coagulation and denaturation of proteins. Moist heat is superior to dry heat in action.

Temperature required to kill microbe by dry heat is more than the moist heat. **Thermal death time** is the minimum time required to kill a suspension of organisms at a predetermined temperature in a specified environment.

Dry Heat Sterilization

It employs higher temperatures in the range of 160 - 180°C and requires exposures time up to 2 hours, depending upon the temperature employed. The benefit of dry heat includes good penetrability and non-corrosive nature which makes it applicable for sterilizing glass wares and metal surgical instruments. It is also used for sterilizing non-aqueous thermostable liquids and thermostable powders.

Dry heat destroys bacterial endotoxins (or pyrogens) which are difficult to eliminate by other means and this property makes it applicable for sterilizing glass bottles which are to be filled aseptically.

Dry Heat Sterilization Methods

Red Heat

Articles such as bacteriological loops, straight wires, tips of forceps and searing spatulas are sterilized by holding them in Bunsen flame till they become red hot. This is a simple method for effective sterilization of such articles, but is limited to those articles that can be heated to redness in flame.

Flaming

This is a method of passing the article over a Bunsen flame, but not heating it to redness. Articles such as scalpels, mouth of test tubes, flasks, glass slides and cover slips are passed through the flame a few times. Even though most vegetative cells are killed, there is no guarantee that spores too would die on such short exposure. This method too is limited to those articles that can be exposed to flame. Cracking of the glassware may occur.

Incineration

This is a method of destroying contaminated material by burning them in incinerator. Articles such as soiled dressings; animal carcasses, pathological material and bedding etc. should be subjected to incineration. This technique results in the loss of the article, hence is suitable only for those articles that have to be disposed. Burning of polystyrene materials emits dense smoke, and hence they should not be incinerated.

Hot Air Oven

This method was introduced by Louis Pasteur. Articles to be sterilized are exposed to high temperature (160°C) for duration of one hour in an electrically heated oven. Since air is poor conductor of heat, even distribution of heat throughout the chamber is achieved by a fan. The heat is transferred to the article by radiation, conduction and convection. The oven should be fitted with a thermostat control, temperature indicator, meshed shelves and must have adequate insulation.

Articles sterilized: Metallic instruments (like forceps, scalpels, scissors), glass wares (such as petri-dishes, pipettes, flasks, all-glass syringes), swabs, oils, grease, petroleum jelly and some pharmaceutical products.

Sterilization process: Articles to be sterilized must be perfectly dry before placing them inside to avoid breakage. Articles must be placed at sufficient distance so as to allow free circulation of air in between. Mouths of flasks, test tubes and both ends of pipettes must be plugged with cotton wool. Articles such as petri dishes and pipettes may be arranged inside metal canisters and then placed. Individual glass articles must be wrapped in Kraft paper or aluminium foils.

Sterilization cycle:

- This takes into consideration the time taken for the articles to reach the sterilizing temperature, maintenance of the sterilizing temperature for a defined period (holding time) and the time taken for the articles to cool down.
- Different temperature-time relations for holding time are
  - 60 minutes at 160°C,
  - 40 minutes at 170°C and
  - 20 minutes at 180°C.
- Increasing temperature by 10 degrees shortens the sterilizing time by 50%.
- The hot air oven must not be opened until the temperature inside has fallen below 60°C to prevent breakage of glassware.

Sterilization control:

Three methods exist to check the efficacy of sterilization process, namely **physical, chemical and biological.**

- **Physical:** Temperature chart recorder and thermocouple.
- **Chemical:** Browne's tube No.3(green spot, color changes from red to green)
- **Biological:** 106 spores of Bacillus subtilis var niger or Clostridium tetany on paper strips are placed inside envelopes and then placed inside the hot air oven.

Upon completion of sterilization cycle, the strips are removed and inoculated into thioglycollate broth or cooked meat medium and incubated at 37°C for 3-5 days.

Proper sterilization should kill the spores and there should not be any growth.

Advantages:

- It is an effective method of sterilization of heat stable articles.

- The articles remain dry after sterilization.
- This is the only method of sterilizing oils and powders.

Disadvantages:

- Since air is poor conductor of heat, hot air has poor penetration.
- Cotton wool and paper may get slightly charred.
- Glasses may become smoky.
- Takes longer time compared to autoclave.

Moist Heat Sterilization

Moist heat sterilization involves the use of steam in the range of 121-134°C. Steam under pressure is used to generate high temperature needed for sterilization. Saturated steam acts as an effective sterilizing agent.

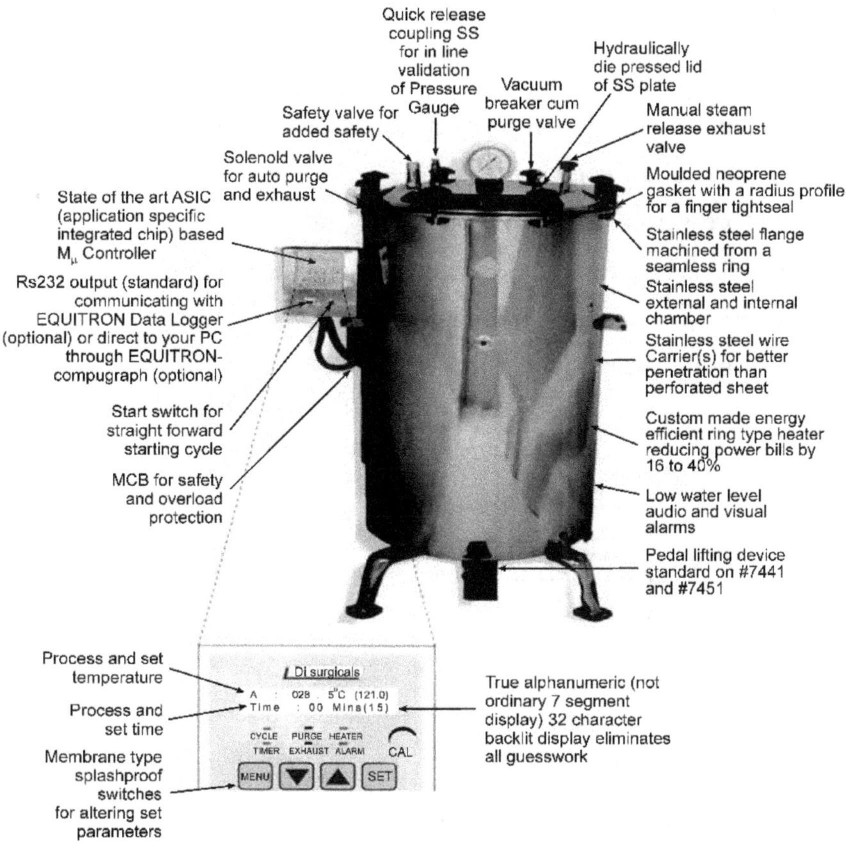

Fig.2.2 Autoclave.

Autoclave

Autoclaves use pressurized steam to destroy microorganisms, and are the most dependable systems available for the decontamination of laboratory waste and the sterilization of laboratory glassware, media, and reagents. For efficient heat transfer, steam must flush the air out of the autoclave chamber. Generally, the conditions employed are Temperature upto121-134°C for 15-20 min under 15 lbs pressure, based on type of material used. Sterilization can be effectively achieved at a temperature above 100°C using an autoclave. Water boils at 100°C at atmospheric pressure, but if pressure is raised, the temperature at which the water boils also increases. In an autoclave the water is boiled in a closed chamber. As the pressure rises, the boiling point of water also raises. At a pressure of 15 lbs inside the autoclave, the temperature is said to be 121°C. Exposure of articles to this temperature for 15 minutes sterilizes them. To destroy the infective agents associated with spongiform encephalopathies (prions), higher temperatures or longer times are used; 135°C or 121°C for at least one hour are recommended.

Advantages of steam:

It has more penetrative power than dry air, it moistens the spores (moisture is essential for coagulation of proteins), condensation of steam on cooler surface releases latent heat, condensation of steam draws in fresh steam.

Different types of autoclave:

- Simple "pressure-cooker type" laboratory autoclave.
- Steam jacketed downward displacement laboratory autoclave.

High pressure pre-vacuum autoclave

Construction and working of Autoclave

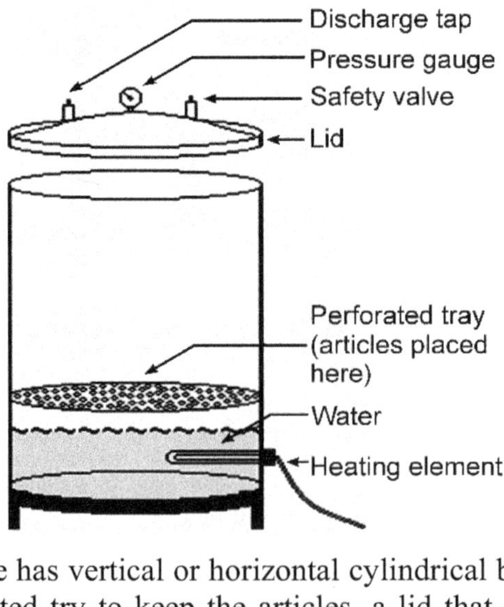

A simple autoclave has vertical or horizontal cylindrical body with a heating element, a perforated try to keep the articles, a lid that can be fastened by screw clamps, a pressure gauge, a safety valve and a discharge tap. The articles to be sterilized must not be tightly packed. The screw caps and cotton plugs must be loosely fitted. The lid is closed but the discharge tap is kept open and the water is heated. As the water starts boiling, the steam drives air out of the discharge tap. When all the air is displaced and steam start appearing through the discharge tap, the tap is closed. The pressure inside is allowed to rise up to 15 lbs per square inch. At this pressure the articles are held for 15 minutes, after which the heating is stopped and the autoclave is allowed to cool. Once the pressure gauge shows the pressure equal to atmospheric pressure, the discharge tap is opened to let the air in.The lid is then opened and articles removed.

Articles sterilized: Culture media, dressings, certain equipment, linen

Precautions:

* Articles should not be tightly packed; the autoclave must not be overloaded.
* Air discharge must be complete and there should not be any residual air trapped inside
* Caps of bottles and flasks should not be tight.
* Autoclave must not be opened until the pressure has fallen or else the contents will boil over.
* Articles must be wrapped in paper to prevent drenching, bottles must not be overfilled.

Merit: Very effective way of sterilization, quicker than hot air oven.

Demerit: Drenching and wetting or articles may occur, trapped air may reduce the efficacy, takes long time to cool.

Radiation Sterilization

Many types of radiation are used for sterilization like electromagnetic radiation (e.g. gamma rays and UV light), particulate radiation (e.g. accelerated electrons). The major target for these radiations is microbial DNA. Radiation sterilization with high energy gamma rays or accelerated electrons has proven to be a useful method for the industrial sterilization of heat sensitive products. Two types of radiation are used, ionizing and non- ionizing.

Non-ionizing rays are low energy rays with poor penetrative power while ionizing rays are high- energy rays with good penetrative power. Since radiation does not generate heat, it is termed "cold sterilization". In some parts of Europe, fruits and vegetables are irradiated to increase their shelf life up to 500 percent.

Non-Ionizing Rays

* Rays of wavelength longer than the visible light are non-ionizing. Microbicidal wavelength of UV rays lie in the range of 200-280 nm, with 260 nm being most effective.
* UV rays are generated using a high-pressure mercury vapor lamp. It is at this wavelength that the absorption by the microorganisms is at its maximum, which results in the germicidal effect.
* UV rays induce formation of thymine-thymine dimers, which ultimately inhibits DNA replication.
* UV readily induces mutations in cells irradiated with a non-lethal dose.
* Microorganisms such as bacteria, viruses, yeast, etc. that are exposed to the effective UV radiation are inactivated within seconds.

Since UV rays don't kill spores, they are considered to be of use in surface disinfection. UV rays are employed to disinfect hospital wards, operation theatres, virus laboratories, corridors, etc.

Disadvantages of using UV rays include low penetrative power, limited life of the UV bulb, some bacteria have DNA repair enzymes that can overcome damage caused by UV rays, organic matter and dust prevents its reach, rays are harmful to skin and eyes. It doesn't penetrate glass, paper or plastic.

Ionizing Rays

Ionizing rays are of two types, particulate and electromagnetic rays. Electron beams are particulate in nature while gamma rays are electromagnetic in nature. High speed electrons are produced by a linear accelerator from a heated cathode. Electron beams are employed to sterilize articles like syringes, gloves, dressing packs, foods and pharmaceuticals. Sterilization is accomplished in few seconds. Unlike electromagnetic rays, the instruments can be switched off. Disadvantage includes poor penetrative power and requirement of sophisticated equipment.

Electromagnetic rays such as gamma rays emanate from nuclear disintegration of certain radioactive isotopes (Co60, Cs137). They have more penetrative power than electron beam but require longer time of exposure. These high-energy radiations damage the nucleic acid of the microorganism. A dosage of 2.5 megarads kills all bacteria, fungi, viruses and spores. It is used commercially to sterilize disposable petri dishes, plastic syringes, antibiotics, vitamins, hormones, glass wares and fabrics. Disadvantages include; unlike electron beams, they can't be switched off, glassware tend to become brownish, loss of tensile strength in fabric.

Gamma irradiation impairs the flavour of certain foods. Bacillus pumilus E601 is used to evaluate sterilization process.

Filtration Sterilization

Filtration does not kill microbes, it separates them out. Membrane filters with pore sizes between 0.2-0.45 μm are commonly used to remove particles from solutions that can't be autoclaved. It is used to remove microbes from heat labile liquids such as serum, antibiotic solutions, sugar solutions, urea solution. Various applications of filtration include removing bacteria from ingredients of culture media, preparing suspensions of viruses and phages free of bacteria, measuring sizes of viruses, separating toxins from culture filtrates, counting bacteria, clarifying fluids and purifying hydrated fluid. Filtration is aided by using either positive or negative pressure using vacuum pumps. The older filters made of earthenware or asbestos are called depth filters.

Different types of filters are

Earthenware filters: These filters are made up of diatomaceous earth or porcelain. They are usually baked into the shape of candle. Different types of earthenware filters are:

a. **Pasteur-Chamberland filter:** These candle filters are from France and are made up of porcelain (sand and kaolin). Similar filter from Britain is Doulton. Chamberland filters are made with various porosities, which are graded as L1, L1a, L2, L3, L5, L7, L9 and L11. Doulton filters are P2, P5 and P11.

b. **Berkefeld filter:** These are made of Kieselguhr, a fossilized diatomaceous earth found in Germany. They are available in three grades depending on their porosity (pore size); they are V (veil), N (normal) and W (wenig).

   Quality of V grade filter is checked using culture suspension of Serrtia marcescens (0.75 μm).

c. **Mandler filter:** This filter is made of kieselguhr, asbestos and plaster of Paris.

   ***Asbestos filters*:** These filters are made from chrysotile type of asbestos, chemically composed of magnesium silicate. They are pressed to form disc, which are to be used only once. The disc is held inside a metal mount, which is sterilized by autoclaving. They are available in following grades; HP/PYR (for removal of pyrogens), HP/EKS (for absolute sterility) and HP/EK (for clarifying).

d. **Sintered glass filters:** These are made from finely ground glass that are fused sufficiently to make small particles adhere to each other. They are usually available in the form of disc fused into a glass funnel. Filters of Grade 5 have average pore diameter of 1-1.5 μm.

   They are washed in running water in reverse direction and cleaned with warm concentrated H_2SO_4 and sterilized by autoclaving.

Membrane filters: These filters are made from a variety of polymeric materials such as cellulose nitrate, cellulose diacetate, polycarbonate and polyester. The older type of membrane, called gradocol (graded colloidion) membrane was composed of cellulose nitrate. Gradocol membranes have average pore diameter of 3-10 μm. The newer ones are composed of cellulose diacetate. These membranes have a pore diameter ranging from 0.015 μm to 12 μm. These filters are sterilized by autoclaving.

Membrane filters are made in two ways, the capillary pore membranes have pores produced by radiation while the labyrinthine pore membranes are produced by forced evaporation of solvents from cellulose esters.

The disadvantages of depth filters are migration of filter material into the filtrate, absorption or retention of certain volume of liquid by the filters, pore sizes are not definite and viruses and mycoplasma could pass through.

The advantages of membrane filters are known porosity, no retention of fluids, reusable after autoclaving and compatible with many chemicals. However, membrane filters have little loading capacity and are fragile.

Air Filters

Air can be filtered using HEPA (High Efficiency Particle Air) filters. They are usually used in biological safety cabinets. HEPA filters are at least 99.97% efficient for removing particles >0.3 μm in diameter. Examples of areas where HEPA filters are used include rooms housing severely neutropenic patients and those operating rooms designated for orthopedic implant procedures.

HEPA filter efficiency is monitored with the dioctylphthalate (DOP) particle test using particles that are 0.3 μm in diameter.

SONIC AND ULTRASONIC VIBRATIONS

Sound waves of frequency >20,000 cycle/second kills bacteria and some viruses on exposing for one hour. Microwaves are not particularly antimicrobial in themselves, rather the killing effect of microwaves are largely due to the heat that they generate. High frequency sound waves disrupt cells.

They are used to clean and disinfect instruments as well as to reduce microbial load. This method is not reliable since many viruses and phages are not affected by these waves.

Filtration Sterilization

Filtration process does not destroy but removes the microorganisms. It is used for both the clarification and sterilization of liquids and gases as it is capable of preventing the passage of both viable and non-viable particles. The major mechanisms of filtration are sieving, adsorption and trapping within the matrix of the filter material. Ex: HEPA FILTERS

Sterilizing grade filters are used in the treatment of heat sensitive injections and ophthalmic solutions, biological products and air and other gases for supply to aseptic areas. They are also used in industry as part of the venting systems on fermenters, centrifuges, autoclaves and freeze driers. Membrane filters are used for sterility testing, there are two types of filters used in filtration sterilization:

(a) Depth filters

(b) **Membrane filters:** These are porous membrane about 0.1 mm thick, made of cellulose acetate, cellulose nitrate, polycarbonate, and polyvinylidene fluoride, or other synthetic material.

CHEMICAL STERILIZATION METHOD

GASEOUS METHOD

The chemically reactive gases such as formaldehyde, (methanol, H.CHO) and ethylene oxide $(CH_2)_2O$ possess biocidal activity. Ethylene oxide is a colourless, odourless, and flammable gas.

The mechanism of antimicrobial action of the two gases is assumed to be through alkylations of sulphydryl, amino, hydroxyl and carboxyl groups on proteins and amino groups of nucleic acids. The concentration ranges (weight of gas per unit chamber volume) are usually in range of 800- 1200 mg/L for ethylene oxide and 15-100 mg/L for formaldehyde with operating temperatures of 45-63°C and 70-75°C respectively. Both of these gases being alkylating agents are potentially mutagenic and carcinogenic. They also produce acute toxicity including irritation of the skin, conjunctiva and nasal mucosa.

Liquid Sterilization (Chemical Method)

Peracetic Acid liquid sterilization: Peracetic acid was found to be sporicidal at low concentrations. It was also found to be water soluble, and left no residue after rinsing. It was also shown to have no harmful health or environmental effects. It disrupts bonds in proteins and enzymes and may also interfere with cell membrane transportation through the rupture of cell walls and may oxidize essential enzymes and impair vital biochemical pathways.

Hydrogen Peroxide Sterilization: This method disperses a hydrogen peroxide solution in a vacuum chamber, creating a plasma cloud. This agent sterilizes by oxidizing key cellular components, which inactivates the microorganisms. The plasma cloud exists only while the energy source is turned on. When the energy source is turned off, water vapour and oxygen are formed, resulting in no toxic residues and harmful emissions. The temperature of this sterilization method is maintained in the 40-50°C range, which makes it particularly well-suited for use with heat-sensitive and moisture-sensitive medical devices. The instruments are wrapped prior to sterilization, and can either be stored or used immediately.

***There are five phases of the hydrogen peroxide processing cycle*:**

i. A vacuum phase creates a vacuum in the chamber and the pressure drops to less than one pound per square inch. This phase lasts about 20 minutes.

ii. In the injection phase, the aqueous hydrogen peroxide is introduced into the vacuum chamber and is vaporized into a gas, which creates a rise in pressure.

iii. During the diffusion phase the hydrogen peroxide vapor spreads throughout the chamber and the increased pressure drives the sterilant into the packs, exposing the instrument surfaces to the sterilant and killing the microorganisms.

iv. During the plasma phase the radio frequency energy is applied, stripping the electrons from some of the molecules and producing a low-temperature plasma cloud. Following this reaction, the activated compounds lose their high energy and recombine to form oxygen and water.

v. The purpose of the venting phase is to introduce filtered air into the chamber and return the chamber to atmospheric pressure so that the door can be opened. It lasts about one minute.

Sterility Indicators

Sterilization procedures should be monitored using biological, Physical, and chemical indicators. Biological indicators, or spore tests, are the most accepted means of monitoring sterilization because they assess the sterilization process directly by killing known highly resistant microorganisms (e.g., *Geobacillus* or *Bacillus* species).

Physical monitoring involves checking the sterilizer gauges, computer displays, or printouts, and documentation in sterilization records that pressure, temperature, and exposure time have reached the levels recommended by the sterilizer manufacturer.

Chemical monitoring uses sensitive chemicals that change colour when exposed to high temperatures or combinations of time and temperature. Examples include chemical indicator tapes, strips, or tabs. Chemical indicator results are obtained immediately following the sterilization cycle and therefore can provide more timely information about the sterilization cycle than a spore test.

A chemical indicator should be used inside every package to verify that the sterilizing agent has penetrated the package and reached the instruments inside. If the internal chemical indicator is not visible from the outside of the package, an external indicator should also be used. Chemical indicators help to differentiate between processed and unprocessed items, eliminating the possibility of using instruments that have not been sterilized.

The two categories of chemical indicators are single-parameter and multiparameter. A single-parameter chemical indicator provides information about only one sterilization parameter (e.g., time or temperature). Multiparameter chemical indicators are designed to react to two or more parameters (e.g., time and temperature or time, temperature, and the presence of steam) and can provide a more reliable indication that sterilization conditions have been met.

DRY HEAT STERILIZATION- STERILITY INDICATORS

Physical indicator: In this process temperature record chart is made of each sterilization cycle with dry heat sterilization. This chart forms the batch documentation and is compared against a master temperature records. The temperature should be taken as the coolest part of the loaded sterilizer, further information on heat distribution and penetration within sterilizer can be gained by the use of thermocouple place at selected site in the chamber or injected into test packs or bottles.

Chemical indicator: It is based on the ability of heat to alter the chemical or physical characteristics of variety of chemical substances. This change should take place only when satisfactory condition for sterilization prevails. Thus, conforming that sterilization cycle has been successfully completed. Chemical indicators generally undergo melting or colour change.

Biological indicator: The biological indicators are the standardized bacterial spore preparations which are usually in the form of suspension in water or culture medium or of spore dried on paper or plastic carriers, they are placed in sterilizer.

After the sterilization process the aqueous suspension /spores are on carriers are aseptically transferred to an appropriate nutrient medium, which is then incubated and occasionally seen for the growth.

Indica-tors	Sterili-zation Methods	Principle	Device	Parameter monitored
Physical	Dry heat	Temperature recording charts	Temperature recording charts	Temperature
Chemical	Dry heat	Temperature sensitive coloured solution	Browne's tube	Temperature, Time
		Temperature sensitive chemical	A temperature sensitive white wax	Temperature

Table contd...

			concealing a black marked	
Biological	Dry heat	Temperature sensitive microbes	Bacillus subtilis	D value

MOIST HEAT STERILIZATION STERILITY INDICATORS

Physical Indicator: Same as that of Dry heat.

Chemical Indicator: Same as that of Dry heat

Biological Indicator: Spores of *G. steareothermophylus* in sealed ampoules of culture medium are used for moist heat sterilization monitoring and these may be incubated directly at 55°C, thus may eliminate the need of aseptic transfer.

Aseptic transfer is also avoided by use of self-contained units where the spores strip and the nutrient medium are present in the same device ready for mixing after use. The bacterial spores should have following qualities; It should be non-pathogenic. Should possess above average resistant to the particular sterilization process.

Indicator	Sterilization	Principle	Device	Parameter monitored
Physical	Moist heat	Temperature recording charts	Temperature recording charts	Temperature
Chemical	Moist heat	Temperature sensitive coloured solution	Browne's tube	Temperature, Time
		Steam sensitive chemical	A device which is impregnated into a carrier material.	Saturated steam
Biological	Moist heat	Temperature sensitive microbes	*Geobacillus stearother-mophilus*	D value

GASEOUS STERILIZATION STERILITY INDICATORS

Physical Indicator: Gas concentration is measured independently of pressure rise, often by reference to weight of gas used.

Chemical Indicator: The chemical indicator used here are Royach Sacket, the indicator paper impregnated with reactive chemical which undergoes a distinct colour change on reaction. Chemical indicators are valuable monitors of the condition prevailing at the coolest of most in accessible part of a sterilizer.

Biological Indicator: As with chemical indicator they are usually packed in dummy packs located at strategic sites in the sterilizer. Alternatively, for gaseous sterilization, these may also be placed in tubular helix device. The species of bacteria generally used for gaseous sterilization are *B.subtilis var.niger* and *B.subtilis var.golbigii*

RADIATION STERILIZATION STERILITY INDICATORS

Physical Indicator: In radiation sterilization a plastic or perspex dosimeter which gradually darkens in proportion to the radiation it absorbs give an accurate measure of the radiation dose and is considered to be the best technique currently available for the radiation sterilization process.

Chemical Indicator: Chemical dosimeter acidified with cerric ammonium sulphate or cerric sulphate solution. These responds to irradiation by dose change in the applied density. Those are considered best and accurately measure relation dose.

Biological Indicator: These consist of standardized bacterial spore preparation which are usually in the form of suspension in water or culture medium or of spore dried on paper or plastic carriers, they are placed in sterilizer. Bacillus pumilus is a **radiation** resistance species. The spores are highly resistant and are **used** to monitor efficiency of **radiation sterilization**.

After the sterilization process the aqueous suspension /spores are on carriers are aseptically transferred to an appropriate nutrient medium, which is then incubated and periodically observed for the growth.

FILTRATION STERILIZATION STERILITY INDICATORS

Physical Indicator: Sterilizing filters are subjected to a bubble point pressure test. This is a technique for determining the pore size of a filter, and may also be used to check the integrity of certain types of filters. The principle of the test is that the wetted filter in its assembled unit is subjected to an increasing air or nitrogen gas pressure difference. The pressure difference recorded when the first bubble of gas breaks away from the filter is related to maximum pore size. When the gas pressure is further increased slowly there is general eruption of bubble over the entire surface. The pressure difference here is related to the mean pore size. Pressure difference below the expected value would signify a damage or faulty filter.

Biological Indicator: Filtration sterilization requires a different approach from biological monitoring, the test effectively measure in the ability of a filter to produce a sterile filtrate from a culture of suitable organism *S. marcesence*, a small gram-negative rod shape bacterium. *B. diminuta* used as a biological indicator having a dimension 0.5 micrometres and 0.3 micrometre respectively has been used for filters of 0.45 micrometre and 0.22 micrometre. The extent of the passage of this organism through membrane filter is enhanced by increasing the filtration pressure. Thus, successful sterile filtration depends markedly on the challenge condition. Such tests are used as the part of filter manufacture characterization and quality assurance process, and user's initial validation procedure.

Moist sterilization by other than Autoclave are Tyndallisation and pasteurization

In practice, Tyndallization was used mostly for food storage. **Tyndallization**, also called fractional sterilization and discontinuous heating, is a form of sterilization that involves boiling goods in cans or jars for about 20 minutes a day, for three days in a row.

Pasteurization, heat-treatment process that destroys pathogenic micro-organisms in certain foods and beverages. It is named for the French scientist Louis Pasteur, who in the 1860s demonstrated that abnormal fermentation of wine and beer could be prevented by heating the beverages to about 57° C (135° F) for a few minutes. Pasteurization of milk, requires temperatures of about 63° C (145° F) maintained for 30 minutes or, alternatively, heating to a higher temperature, 72° C (162° F), and holding for 15 seconds (and yet higher temperatures for shorter periods of time). The times and temperatures are those determined to be necessary to destroy the Mycobacterium tuberculosis and other more heat-resistant of the non-spore-forming, disease-causing microorganisms found in milk. The treatment also destroys most of the microorganisms that cause spoilage and so prolongs the storage time of food.

UNIT III

Fungi and Viruses

Fungi

Fungi, latin for mushroom, are eukaryotes which are responsible for decomposition and nutrient cycling through the environment. The kingdom Fungi includes an enormous variety of living organisms collectively referred to as Ascomycota, or true Fungi. Fungi are not capable of photosynthesis: they are heterotrophic because they use complex organic compounds as sources of energy and carbon. Some fungal organisms multiply only asexually, whereas others undergo both asexual reproduction and sexual reproduction. Most fungi produce a large number of spores, which are haploid cells that can undergo mitosis to form multicellular, haploid individuals. Like bacteria, fungi play an essential role in ecosystems because they are decomposers and participate in the cycling of nutrients by breaking down organic and inorganic materials to simple molecules.

Fungi often interact with other organisms, forming beneficial or mutualistic associations. For example, most terrestrial plants form symbiotic relationships with fungi. The roots of the plant connect with the underground parts of the fungus forming mycorrhizae. Through mycorrhizae, the fungus and plant exchange nutrients and water, greatly aiding the survival of both species. Alternatively, lichens are an association between a fungus and its photosynthetic partner (usually an alga). Fungi also cause serious infections in plants and animals. In humans, fungal infections are generally considered challenging to treat. Unlike bacteria, fungi do not respond to traditional antibiotic therapy because they are eukaryotes. Fungi have many commercial applications. The food industry uses yeasts in baking, brewing, and cheese and wine making. Many industrial compounds are by products of fungal fermentation. Fungi are the source of many commercial enzymes and antibiotics.

Fungi Cell Structure and Function

Fungi are unicellular or multicellular thick-cell-walled heterotroph decomposers that eat decaying matter and make tangles of filaments.

Fungi are eukaryotes and have a complex cellular organization. As eukaryotes, fungal cells contain a membrane-bound nucleus where the DNA is wrapped around histone proteins. A few types of fungi have structures comparable to bacterial plasmids (loops of DNA). Fungal cells also contain mitochondria and a complex system of internal membranes, including the endoplasmic reticulum and Golgi apparatus.

Unlike plant cells, fungal cells do not have chloroplasts or chlorophyll. Many fungi display bright colours arising from other cellular pigments, ranging from red to green to black. The poisonous *Amanita muscaria* (fly agaric) is recognizable by its bright red cap with white patches. Pigments in fungi are associated with the cell wall. They play a protective role against ultraviolet radiation and can be toxic.

The rigid layers of fungal cell walls contain complex polysaccharides called chitin and glucans. Chitin, also found in the exoskeleton of insects, gives structural strength to the cell walls of fungi. The wall protects the cell from desiccation and predators. Fungi have plasma membranes similar to other eukaryotes, except that the structure is stabilized by ergosterol: a steroid molecule that replaces the cholesterol found in animal cell membranes. Most members of the kingdom Fungi are nonmotile.

Growth

The vegetative body of a fungus is a unicellular or multicellular thallus. Dimorphic fungi can change from the unicellular to multicellular state depending on environmental conditions. Unicellular fungi are generally referred to as yeasts. *Saccharomyces cerevisiae* (baker's yeast) and *Candida* species (the agents of thrush, a common fungal infection) are examples of unicellular fungi.

Most fungi are multicellular organisms. They display two distinct morphological stages: the vegetative and reproductive. The vegetative stage consists of a tangle of slender thread-like structures called hyphae (singular, hypha), whereas the reproductive stage can be more conspicuous. The mass of hyphae is a mycelium. It can grow on a surface, in soil or decaying material, in a liquid, or even on living tissue. Although individual hyphae must be observed under a microscope, the mycelium of a fungus can be very large, with some species truly being "the fungus humongous." The giant *Armillaria solidipes* (honey mushroom) is considered the largest organism on Earth, spreading across more than 2,000 acres of underground soil in eastern Oregon; it is estimated to be at least 2,400 years old.

Most fungal hyphae are divided into separate cells by endwalls called septa (singular, septum). In most phyla of fungi, tiny holes in the septa allow for the rapid flow of nutrients and small molecules from cell to cell along the hypha.

They are described as perforated septa. The hyphae in bread moulds (which belong to the Phylum Zygomycota) are not separated by septa. Instead, they are formed by large cells containing many nuclei, an arrangement described as coenocytic hyphae. Fungi thrive in environments that are moist and slightly acidic; they can grow with or without light.

Nutrition

Like animals, fungi are heterotrophs: they use complex organic compounds as a source of carbon, rather than fix carbon dioxide from the atmosphere as do some bacteria and most plants. In addition, fungi do not fix nitrogen from the atmosphere. Like animals, they must obtain it from their diet. However, unlike most animals, which ingest food and then digest it internally in specialized organs, fungi perform these steps in the reverse order: digestion precedes ingestion. First, exoenzymes are transported out of the hyphae, where they process nutrients in the environment. Then, the smaller molecules produced by this external digestion are absorbed through the large surface area of the mycelium.

Fungi are mostly saprobes (saprophyte is an equivalent term): organisms that derive nutrients from decaying organic matter. They obtain their nutrients from dead or decomposing organic matter, mainly plant material. Fungal exoenzymes are able to break down insoluble polysaccharides, such as the cellulose and lignin of dead wood, into readily-absorbable glucose molecules. The carbon, nitrogen, and other elements are thus released into the environment. Because of their varied metabolic pathways, fungi fulfil an important ecological role and are being investigated as potential tools in bioremediation.

Some fungi are parasitic, infecting either plants or animals. Smut and Dutch elm disease affect plants, whereas athlete's foot and candidiasis (thrush) are medically important fungal infections in humans.

Fungi Reproduction

Fungi can reproduce asexually by fragmentation, budding, or producing spores, or sexually with homothallic or heterothallic mycelia.

Fungi reproduce sexually and/or asexually. Perfect fungi reproduce both sexually and asexually, while imperfect fungi reproduce only asexually (by mitosis).

In both sexual and asexual reproduction, fungi produce spores that disperse from the parent organism by either floating on the wind or hitching a ride on an animal. Fungal spores are smaller and lighter than plant seeds. The giant puffball mushroom bursts open and releases trillions of spores. The huge number of spores released increases the likelihood of landing in an environment that will support growth.

Asexual Reproduction

Fungi reproduce asexually by fragmentation, budding, or producing spores. Fragments of hyphae can grow new colonies. Mycelial fragmentation occurs when a fungal mycelium separates into pieces with each component growing into a separate mycelium. Somatic cells in yeast form buds. During budding (a type of cytokinesis), a bulge forms on the side of the cell, the nucleus divides mitotically, and the bud ultimately detaches itself from the mother cell.

The most common mode of asexual reproduction is through the formation of asexual spores, which are produced by one parent only (through mitosis) and are genetically identical to that parent. Spores allow fungi to expand their distribution and colonize new environments. They may be released from the parent thallus, either outside or within a special reproductive sac called a sporangium.

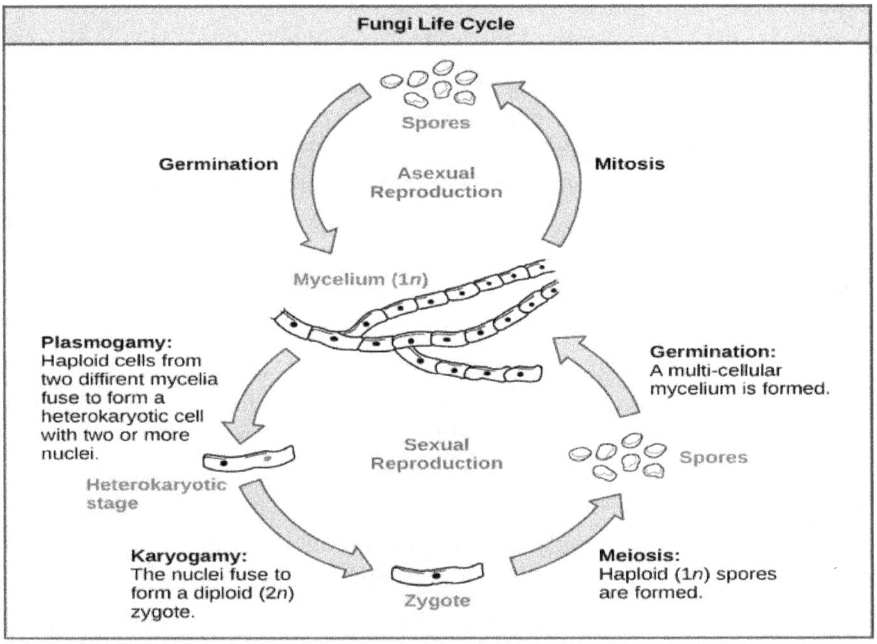

Fig 3.1. Fungi Life style.

There are many types of asexual spores. Conidiospores are unicellular or multicellular spores that are released directly from the tip or side of the hypha. Other asexual spores originate in the fragmentation of a hypha to form single cells that are released as spores; some of these have a thick wall surrounding the fragment. Yet others bud off the vegetative parent cell. Sporangiospores are produced in a sporangium.

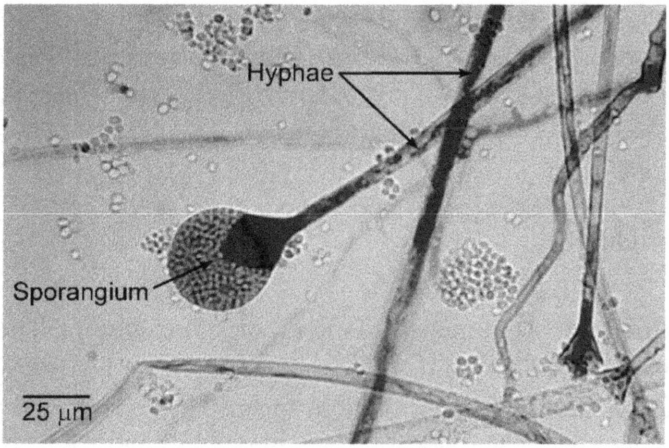

Fig 3.2. Release of spores from a sporangium.

This bright field light micrograph shows the release of spores from a sporangium at the end of a hypha called a sporangiophore. The organism depicted is a Mucor sp. fungus: a mould often found indoors.

Sexual Reproduction

Sexual reproduction introduces genetic variation into a population of fungi. In fungi, sexual reproduction often occurs in response to adverse environmental conditions. Two mating types are produced. When both mating types are present in the same mycelium, it is called homothallic, or self-fertile. Heterothallic mycelia require two different, but compatible, mycelia to reproduce sexually.

Although there are many variations in fungal sexual reproduction, all include the following three stages. First, during plasmogamy (literally, "marriage or union of cytoplasm"), two haploid cells fuse, leading to a dikaryotic stage where two haploid nuclei coexist in a single cell. During karyogamy ("nuclear marriage"), the haploid nuclei fuse to form a diploid zygote nucleus. Finally, meiosis takes place in the gametangia (singular, gametangium) organs, in which gametes of different mating types are generated. At this stage, spores are disseminated into the environment.

Characteristics of Fungi

1. Fungi are eukaryotic organisms means they have true nucleus which are enclosed in membranes.
2. They are non-vascular organisms. They do not have vascular system. Xylem and Phloem are absent.

3. Fungi have cell walls (plants also have cell walls, but animals have no cell walls).
4. There is no embryonic stage for fungi.
5. They reproduce by means of spores. There are sexual and asexual spores. Sexual spores are Oospores, Zygospores, Ascospores, Basidiospores, etc. and Asexual spores are Sporangiospores, Aplanospores, Zoospores, Conidia, etc.
6. Depending on the species and conditions both sexual and asexual spores may be produced.
7. They are typically non-motile.
8. Fungi exhibit the phenomenon of alteration of generation. They have both haploid and diploid stage.
9. Fungi are achlorophyllous, which means they lack the chlorophyll pigments present in the chloroplasts in plant cells and which are necessary for photosynthesis.
10. The vegetative body of the fungi may be unicellular or composed of microscopic threads called hyphae.
11. Hyphae can grow and form a network called a mycelium.
12. Yeasts are unicellular fungi that do not produce hyphae.

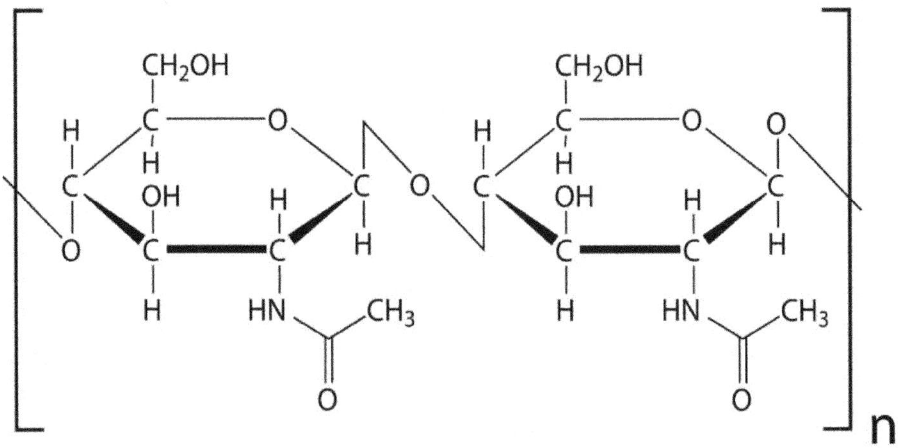

Fig 3.3. Structure of Chitin.

13. The structure of cell wall is similar to plants but chemically the fungi cell wall is composed of chitin (C8H13O5N) n.
14. The cell membrane of a fungus has a unique sterol and ergosterol.
15. Fungi are heterotrophic organisms. They obtain its food and energy from organic substances, plant and animal matters.

16. Fungi grow best in acidic environment (tolerate acidic pH).
17. Fungi digest the food first and then ingest the food, to accomplish this the fungi produce exoenzymes like Hydrolases, Lyases, Oxidoreductase, Transferase, etc.
18. Fungi store their food as starch.
19. Biosynthesis of chitin occurs in fungi.
20. Many of the fungi have a small nucleus with repetitive DNA.
21. During mitosis the nuclear envelope is not dissolved.
22. Nutrition in fungi – they are saprophytes (gets energy from dead and decaying matters), or parasites (lives in a host, attack and kill)or symbionts (mutually beneficial).
23. Optimum temperature of growth for most saprophytic fungi is

    20- 30°C while (30-37) °C for parasitic fungi.
24. Growth rate of fungi is slower than that of bacteria.
25. Reproduction in fungi is both by sexual and asexual means.
26. Sexual state is referred to as teleomorph (fruiting body), asexual

    state is referred to as anamorph (mould like).
27. Reproduction occurs by both asexual (Axamorph) and sexual (Teliomorph) mode:

    Asexual methods: fragmentation, fsomatic budding, fission, asexual spore formation.

    Sexual methods: gametic copulation, gamate-gametangium opulation, gametangium copulation, somatic copulation and Spermatization.
28. Pheromone is a chemical substance produced by fungi, which leads to the sexual reproduction between male &female fungi cells.
29. Some fungi are macroscopic and can be seen by naked eyes.

    Mold or mushrooms are examples of macroscopic form of fungi.
30. Only about 300 species of fungi are infectious to human.

    Examples: *Candida albicans, Aspergillus, Blastomyces, Coccidioides, Cryptococcus neoformans, Histoplasma, Pneumocystis jirovecii.*

Classification of Fungi

The nomenclature is binomial, with a generic and a specific name (eg: *Aspergillus niger*). Species are collected in general, genera in families (suffix – aceae), families in orders (suffix-ales), and orders in classes (suffix-mycetes).

The division of mycota, or fungi and moulds, includes the true slime moulds (Myxomycetes), the lower fungi (Phycomycetes), and the higher fungi (Eumycetes).

Alexopolous and Mims proposed fungal classification in 1979. They place the fungi including the slime molds in the kingdom mycetae of the super kingdom Eukaryota which, in addition, includes four other kingdoms.

- They divide the kingdom mycetae into **three** divisions namely:
    1. Gymnomycota
    2. Mastigomycota and
    3. Amastigomycota
- The division is subdivided into subdivision, classes, sub-classes, and orders.

Division I Gymnomycota

- It includes phagotrophic organism devoid of cell walls.
- This division comprises two subdivisions.
- These are Acrasiogymnomycotina and Plasmodiogynomycotina.

Subdivision 1. Acrasiogymnomycotina

It includes a single class Acrasiomycetes.

Class 1. Acrasiomycetes

- Lacks flagellated cells except for one species. The class comprises two subclasses.
- Acrasiomycetidae and Dictyosteliomycetidae.

Subdivision 2. Plasmodiogymnomycotina

It is divided into two classes:

Class 1 Protosteliomycetes

Class 2 Mycomycetes

It includes the true slime mold and comprises three sub class namely:

Sub Class 1. Ceratiomyxomycomycetidae

Order – Ceratiomyxales

Sub Class 2. Mycogasteomycetidae

It comprises of four orders.

Order -

1. Liceales
2. Echinosteleales
3. Trichlales
4. Physarales

Sub Class 3. Stemonitomycetidae

Order 1. Stemonitales

Division II Mastigomycota

- Includes fungi with absorptive nutrition, unicellular or filamentous, mycelium coemocytic.
- It comprises two sub divisions:

Sub division 1 Haplomastigomycotina

- Includes fungi with uni-or, bi-flagellate zoospores.

Class 1 Chytridiomycetes– Fungi producing zoospores furnished with a single whiplash flagellum inserted at the posterior end.

Class 2 Hyphochytridiomycetes- Motile cells with a single tinsel flagellum inserted at the anterior end.

Class 3 Plasmodiophoromycetes- Parasitic fungi producing biflagellate motile cells with both the flagella of whiplash type inserted at the anterior end.

Sub division 2. Diplomastigomycotima Sexual reproduction ooagamous, zoospores biflagellate.

Class 1 Oomycetes

It comprises four orders:

Order 1 Lagenidiales

Order 2 Saprolegnailes

Order 3. Leptomitales

Order 4. Peronosporales

Division III Amastigomycota

Fungi with absorptive nutrition, motile cells lacking, mycelium aseptate or septate.

This includes four sub divisions:

Sub division 1 Zygomycotina

Class 1 Zygomycetes – it includes six orders.

Class 2 Trichomycetes – it comprises five orders.

Sub division 2 Ascomycotina

Fungi usually with a septate mycelium producing haploid ascospores in sac like cells called asci.

Class 1 Ascomycetes- divided into five sub classes:

Sub class 1. Hemiascomycetidae- comprising three orders.

Sub class 2. Plectomycetidae- Five orders

Sub class 3. Hymenoascomycetidae – Ten orders

Sub class 4 Laboulbeniomycetidae – Two orders

Sub class 5 Lowloascomycetidae – five orders

Sub division 3. Basidiomycotina

Septate mycelium, produces basidiospores, exogenously on various types of basidia.

Class 1 Basidiomycetes: it is split into 3 sub clases:

Sub class 1 Holobasidiomycetidae

Sub class 2 Phragmobasidiomycetidae

Sub class 3 Teliomycetidae

Sub division 4. Deuteromycotina

It includes imperfect fungi in which sexual stage is unknown. It comprises a single form class.

Form Class Deuteromycetes with three form sub classes namely Blastomycetidae, Coelomycetidae and Hyphomycetidae.

On the Basis of Spore Production

On the basis of the organization of the vegetative thallus, the morphology of reproductive structures, the way of spores production and particular life cycle involved the kingdom mycota is classified into following divisions.

Phycomycetes

- It includes the simplest type of fungi. It is also called as Algae-Fungi because most of the characteristics of them are similar to algae like Vaucheria.

- They have simple thallus which is unicellular or coenocytic or aseptate filaments.
- They reproduce asexually by the formation of zoospores or non-motile spores.
- Sexual reproduction is isogamous or heterogamous which takes place by game tangial contact.
- The diploid phase is represented by zygote.
- Phycomycetes has been classified into subclasses: oomycetes and zygomycetes.

Oomycetes

- Oomycetes range from a primitive unicellular thallus to a profusely branched filamentous mycelium.
- Many members of them are terrestrial and obligate parasites.
- Asexually they reproduce by biflagellate zoospores.
- Sexual reproduction is oogamy that involves the fusion of male and female gametes to form oospore.
- Oospore undergoes meiosis to produce haploid biflagellate zoospores.
- Example: Phytophthora infestans (causes potato blight)

Zygomycetes

- The group is named zygomycetes because a diploid resting spore called the zygospore is formed during the life cycle.
- They are mostly saprophytic; some others are parasites on plants and animals.
- The vegetative body is mycelium which is well developed, profusely branched and coenocytic.
- The absence of motile sexual or asexual cells.
- The asexual reproduction takes place by sporangiospores, aplanospores or by conidia.
- Sexual reproduction occurs by conjugation of gametangia resulting in the formation of zygospore.
- Examples; Rhizopus, Mucor etc.

Ascomycetes

- The species of ascomycetes are called the sac fungi because they produce sexual pores within the sac-like vascus.
- General Characteristics

- Ascomycetes are mostly terrestrial occurring as saprophytes or parasites.
- They have well-developed, branched, septate mycelium except yeast. Yeast is a unicellular fungus.
- Asexually they reproduce by non-motile spores, conidia, oidia or chlamydospores.
- Sexual reproduction takes place by the fusion of gametangia of opposite mating types.
- There is absence of motile cells.
- Examples, Saccharomyces cerevisiae, Penicillium, Aspergillus etc.

Basidiomycetes

- The members of basidiomycetes are saprophytic or parasitic. The group is named basidiomycetes as they produce the basidiospores at the club-shaped basidium during sexual reproduction.
- Mycelium is highly developed, profusely branched and septate.
- The mycelia are differentiated into two mating types; (+ve) and (-ve).
- There are two kinds of mycelium; primary mycelium and secondary mycelium.
- Asexual reproduction takes place by fragmentation, budding, oidia, conidia or chlamydospore.
- The dikaryotic cell is formed during sexual reproduction.
- The absence of motile cell throughout the life cycle.
- Basidiomycetes are the most advanced fungi as their fructifications are often large and prominent.
- Examples; Mushrooms, Puccinia, Ustilago etc.

Deuteromycetes (The Imperfect Fungi)

- Deuteromycetes compromises more than 17000 species of the diverse habits and habitats. It is considered as an artificial class of fungi.
- The fungi are saprophytes as well as parasites. Parasitic fungi cause serious diseases to plants, animals including human beings.
- Some of them are unicellular while others are multicellular.
- They reproduce asexually by conidia along with some other types of spores.
- The sexual reproduction is entirely absent.
- The asexual stage or imperfect stage in Deuteromycetes is well defined. But the sexual or perfect stage is absent in life cycle, therefore, they are called 'Fungi Imperfecti'.

- Example; Alternaria, Fusarium, Helminthosporium etc.

Classification of Medically Important Fungi

Classification Based on Site

Mycoses are classified as superficial, cutaneous, subcutaneous, or systemic (deep) infections depending on the type and degree of tissue involvement and the host response to the pathogen.

Superficial mycoses (or **tineas**) mostly occur in the tropics and are restricted to the outer surface of the hair and skin. Examples are:

- *Piedraia hortae*, a filamentous member of the Ascomycota which causes black piedra, a disease of the hair shaft characterised by brown/black nodules on the scalp hair (actually the ascostromata of the fungus).
- *Trichosporon cutaneum*, a yeast belonging to the Basidiomycota that is common in soil, water samples, plants, mammals and birds, as well as being a member of the normal flora of mouth, skin and nails. It causes white piedra, a superficial infection of the skin, and scalp and pubic hair (although it is emerging as an opportunistic pathogen of the immuno compromised).

Cutaneous mycoses. There are three genera of fungi that commonly cause disease in the non-living tissues of skin, hair, or nails/claws of people and animals, by growing in a zone just above where the protein keratin is deposited.

These three genera are *Microspore*, *Trichophyton* and *Epidermophyton* (all filamentous Ascomycota) and they are often labelled 'dermatophytes' (with the disease being called 'dermatophytosis') although, of course, they are not plants, so they can't be any sort of '-phyte' and a better term would be dermatomycosis. These fungi all have the ability to degrade keratin and grow as non-invasive saprotrophs on skin and its appendages, but their growth causes irritation and inflammation of underlying epithelial cells, this being an allergic reaction that may result in death of these cells.

Subcutaneous mycoses are generally caused by fungi that are normally saprotrophic inhabitants of soil, particularly in tropical and subtropical areas of Africa, India and South America, which become infective by being introduced through wounds in the skin. Most infections involve people who normally walk barefoot.

- *Madurella mycetomatis* and *M. grisea* (filamentous, Ascomycota) cause human **mycetoma** (common name: madura foot), which is a localised infection causing locally invasive tumour-like abscesses, accompanied by chronic inflammation, resulting in swelling, distortion and ulceration of the infected body part. The fungus is introduced through mild wounds in the skin and may grow for several years in the cutaneous and subcutaneous tissues, extending to connective tissues and bones. Mycetomas are usually resistant to chemotherapy, leaving surgery, even amputation, as the only resolution.

- *Sporothrix schenckii* (thermally dimorphic, Ascomycota) causes **sporotrichosis.** *Sporothrix* is the anamorph and *Ophiostoma stenoceras* the teleomorph. The fungus occurs in soil worldwide although the disease is localised, with Peru having the highest prevalence of *Sporothrix schenckii* infections. Also called 'rose handler's disease', sporotrichosis starts by entry of the fungus through minor skin injury and can then spread through the lymphatic system. The fungus is dimorphic, forming septate vegetative hyphae, conidiophores and conidia at 25°C, while at 37°C oval to cigar-shaped budding yeast cells are produced. As the yeast form is distributed by the lymphatic system, disseminated sporotrichosis can result in infections of the lungs and bones and joints, endophthalmitis (inflammation of the internal layers of the eye), meningitis and invasive sinusitis.

Systemic mycoses are infections that affect the whole body. We divide these into mycoses due to primary (usually dimorphic) virulent pathogens, and those due to opportunistic pathogens.

Classification Based on Route of Acquisition

- Infecting fungi may be either exogenous or endogenous.
- When classified according to the route of acquisition, a fungal infection may be designated as exogenous or endogenous in origin.
- If classified as exogenous, an infecting organism may be transmitted by airborne, cutaneous, or percutaneous routes.
- An endogenously-acquired fungal infection may be acquired from colonization or reactivation of a fungus from latent infection.

Classification Based on Virulence

Primary pathogens can establish infections in normal hosts. Opportunistic pathogens cause disease in individuals with compromised host defense mechanisms.

- Deep mycoses are caused by primary pathogenic and opportunistic fungal pathogens.
- The primary pathogenic fungi are able to establish infection in a normal host; whereas, opportunistic pathogens require a compromised host in

order to establish infection (e.g., cancer, organ transplantation, surgery, and AIDS).

- The primary deep pathogens usually gain access to the host via the respiratory tract. Opportunistic fungi causing deep mycosis invade via the respiratory tract, alimentary tract, or intravascular devices.
- The primary systemic fungal pathogens include *Coccidioides immitis, Histoplasma capsulatum, Blastomyces dermatitidis*, and *Paracoccidioides brasiliensis*.
- The opportunistic fungal pathogens include Cryptococcus neoformans, Candida, Aspergillusspp., Penicillium marneffei, the Zygomycetes, Trichosporon beigelii, and Fusarium spp.

Fungal culture

The most direct and usually conclusive means of establishing the diagnosis of a fungal infection is to grow the fungus from a patient sample. Numerous different samples can yield a fungus, including blood, cerebrospinal fluid, pus, urine, tissue, respiratory samples (sputum, bronchoscopy lavage), pleural, pericardial or peritoneal fluid, skin scraping, hair, nail clippings, oral or vaginal samples. Processing of these samples may involve centrifugation or softening/liquidisation to allow spreading of the sample onto an agar medium. A number of laboratory manuals and specific describe the methods for doing this although remarkably few comparative studies comparing one method with another have been done.

The importance of media selection

The yield of most fungi is improved by direct culture of samples on so-called 'fungal media'. For some fungi, cultures are always or almost always negative on bacterial media, examples being *Histoplasma*, Mucorales and *Coccidioides* spp. The culture of *Aspergillus* spp. on bacterial media is ~30% less effective than on fungal media.

General purpose media that are commonly used for fungal culture are Sabouraud dextrose, malt extract and less commonly brain heart infusion medium. To prevent contamination of the medium by bacteria, chloramphenicol is used, but prevents the growth of *Actinomyces*, which others grows well on Sabouraud dextrose agar. For reducing the frequency of environmental fungal growth, cycloheximide is added, but this reduces the yield of many opportunistic fungi including *Aspergillus* spp., *Cryptococcus neoformans* and Mucorales isolates. Therefore, if cycloheximide is used, one agar plate not containing it should also be used in parallel.

Media for selective culture and presumptive identification

There are some additional specialised media that can be used directly on specimens to allow separation of similar looking colonies including bird seed agar to identify *Cryptococcus* spp. in respiratory cultures from HIV patients or chromogenic agar for the direct, partial identification of *Candida* spp.

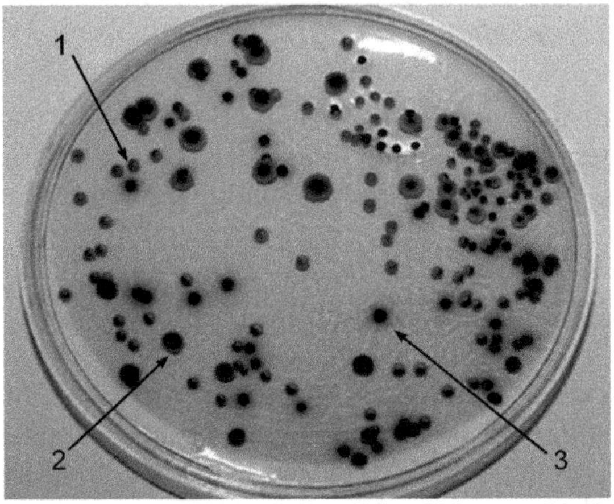

ChromAgar is used to identify : 1=Candida albicans; 2= Candida krusei; 3=Candida tropicalis

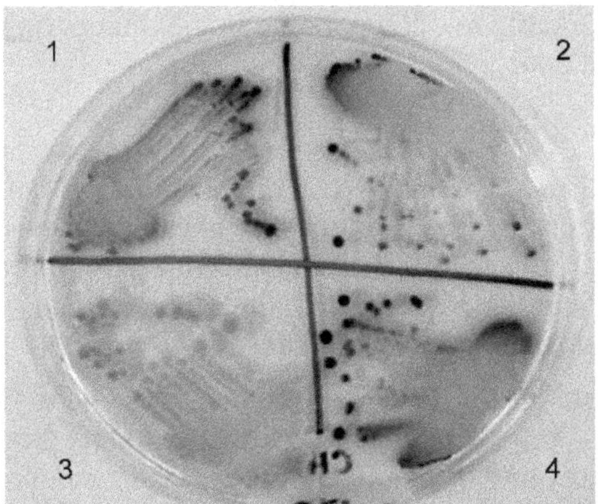

ChromAgar :1=C glabrata; 2= C albicans 3=C krusei; 4=C tropicalis

Fig 3.4. ChromAgar Plates.

Blood culture for fungi

Numerous blood culture systems have been used, including 'standard' bacterial cultures and more specialised systems such as the lysis centrifugation system, the Septi-Check systems, and special bottles within an automated system (sometimes of Mycobacteria and fungi). A small number of comparisons have been done of these systems, and the choice matters a great deal more when the range of potential infecting fungi includes *Cryptococcus neoformans*, *Histoplasma capsulatum* and *Penicillium marneffei*. In current automated blood culture systems, *Candida glabrata* grows more slowly and much more often in the anaerobic bottle, so both aerobic and anaerobic bottles should be filled with blood. The yield from blood culture is higher if patients are not taking antifungal agents[2] and if at least 20mL of blood is cultured.

Incubation conditions

The standard temperature for incubation of fungi is 30°C and cultures should be incubated in a humidified environment for 21 days. They should be inspected daily for at least a week, and at least 3 times weekly thereafter. Some fungi are very slow to grow, notably *Histoplasma* spp., and may need longer incubation times. Culture of respiratory cultures at 42°C prevents the growth of *Candida* spp. allowing *Aspergillus* spp. to flourish without competition.

Handling growth and procedures for identification

Once colonies are visible, they should be inspected carefully for their morphology. Yeasts can be further identified by their growth pattern on specialised media such as cornmeal agar and with biochemistry testing. Some presumptive identification of yeasts can be made based on colour and colony morphology on chromogenic media. Some rapid testing systems are available which are more or less comprehensive and reliable. Published comparisons of these methodologies are available.

Filamentous fungi are harder to identify. Without spores or other sterile structures, the only real distinction that can be made is whether the hyphae are septate or not (i.e. are likely be Mucorales, *Basidiobolus ranarum* or *Conidiobolus* spp. Media that can assist with sporulation include potato dextrose agar. If the colony will not spore, only molecular identification is possible. Once the colony has sporulated identification by microscopy using phenol cotton blue or another simple means of highlighting the distinctive structures of the fungus allows an experienced mycologist to identify to at least genus level in the vast majority of cases. Species identification of filamentous fungi can be very difficult or impossible without additional data such as colour and morphology of additional media, differential temperature growth rates and molecular information

Fungal Infections

Of the estimated 2 million species of fungi on earth about 600 have caused disease. Most infections are caused by the genera *Trichophyton, Candida,*

Aspergillus and Cryptococcus. Other relatively common genera causing infection include Microsporum, Malassezia, Histoplasma, Coccidioides and Pneumocystis. Common genera causing allergic fungal disease include *Aspergillus, Alternaria, Cladosporium, Malassezia and Penicillium.*

Fungal infections are best sub-divided into 5 groups, although there are some overlaps. Most serious fungal infections are 'hidden', occurring as a consequence of other health problems such as asthma, AIDS, cancer, transplantation and corticosteroid therapies. Infections are grouped as follows in order of broadly decreasing severity:

- Invasive fungal infections which are often fatal (esp. cryptococcal meningitis, invasive aspergillosis, Candida bloodstream infection, Pneumocystis pneumonia).
- Chronic lung or deep tissue infection (esp. chronic pulmonary aspergillosis)
- Allergic fungal disease (esp. allergic bronchopulmonary aspergillosis (ABPA), severe asthma with fungal sensitisation (SAFS))
- Mucosal infection (esp. oral and oesophageal candidiasis, Candida vaginitis (thrush))
- Skin, hair and nail infection (esp. ringworm, tinea capitis, athlete's foot, onychomycosis).

The Importance of Fungi

They are important in an enormous variety of ways.

- **Recycling**

Fungi, together with bacteria, are responsible for most of the recycling which returns dead material to the soil in a form in which it can be reused. Without fungi, these recycling activities would be seriously reduced. We would effectively be lost under piles many metres thick, of dead plant and animal remains.

- **Mycorrhizae and plant growth**

Fungi are vitally important for the good growth of most plants, including crops, through the development of mycorrhizal associations. As plants are at the base of most food chains, if their growth was limited, all animal life, including human, would be seriously reduced through starvation.

- **Food**

Fungi are also important directly as food for humans. Many mushrooms are edible and different species are cultivated for sale worldwide. While this is a very small proportion of the actual food that we eat, fungi are also widely used in the production of many foods and drinks. These include cheeses, beer and wine, bread, some cakes, and some soya bean products.

While a great many wild fungi are edible, it can be difficult to correctly identify them. Some mushrooms are deadly if they are eaten. Fungi with names such as 'Destroying Angel' and 'Death Cap' give us some indication that it would not be a terribly good idea to eat them! In some countries, collecting wild mushrooms to eat is a popular activity. It is always wise to be totally sure that what you have collected is edible and not a poisonous look-a-like.

- **Medicines**

Penicillin, perhaps the most famous of all antibiotic drugs, is derived from a common fungus called *Penicillium.* Many other fungi also produce antibiotic substances, which are now widely used to control diseases in human and animal populations. The discovery of antibiotics revolutionized health care worldwide.

Some fungi which parasitise caterpillars have also been traditionally used as medicines. The Chinese have used a particular caterpillar fungus as a tonic for hundreds of years. Certain chemical compounds isolated from the fungus may prove to be useful treatments for certain types of cancer.

A fungus which parasitises Rye crops causes a disease known as Ergot. The fungus can occur on a variety of grasses. It produces small hard structures, known as sclerotia. These sclerotia can cause poisoning in humans and animals which have eaten infected material. However, these same sclerotia are also the source of a powerful and important drug which has uses in childbirth.

- **Biocontrol**

Fungi such as the Chinese caterpillar fungus, which parasitise insects, can be extremely useful for controlling insect pests of crops. The spores of the fungi are sprayed on the crop pests. Fungi have been used to control Colorado potato beetles, which can devastate potato crops. Spittlebugs, leaf hoppers and citrus rust mites are some of the other insect pests which have been controlled using fungi. This method is generally cheaper and less damaging to the environment than using chemical pesticides.

- **Crop Diseases**

Fungal parasites may be useful in biocontrol, but they can also have enormous negative consequences for crop production. Some fungi are parasites of plants. Most of our common crop plants are susceptible to fungal attack of one kind or another. Spore production and dispersal is enormously efficient in fungi and plants of the same species crowded together in fields are ripe for attack. Fungal diseases can on occasion result in the loss of entire crops if they are not treated with antifungal agents.

- **Animal Disease**

Fungi can also parasitise domestic animals causing diseases, but this is not usually a major economic problem. A wide range of fungi also live on and in humans, but most coexist harmlessly. Athletes foot and Candida infections are examples of human fungal infections.

- **Food Spoilage**

It has already been noted that fungi play a major role in recycling organic material. The fungi which make our bread and jam go mouldy are only recycling organic matter, even though in this case, we would prefer that it didn't happen! Fungal damage can be responsible for large losses of stored food, particularly food which contains any moisture. Dry grains can usually be stored successfully, but the minute they become damp, moulds are likely to render them inedible. This is obviously a problem where large quantities of food are being produced seasonally and then require storage until they are needed.

Virus

Viruses are small obligate intracellular parasites, which by definition contain either a RNA or DNA genome surrounded by a protective, virus-coded protein coat. A complete virus particle is called a virion. It has the smallest size in the microorganisms **20-300nm.**They lack essential metabolic machinery to synthesize their own essential proteins hence has to depend on the hosts. Viruses hence are called **obligate intracellular parasites**. They lack nucleus, cytoplasm, cell membrane and other cellular components.

The main function of the virion is to deliver its DNA or RNA genome into the host cell so that the genome can be expressed (transcribed and translated) by the host cell. The viral genome, often with associated basic proteins, is packaged inside a symmetric protein capsid. The nucleic acid-associated protein, called nucleoprotein, together with the genome, forms the nucleocapsid. In enveloped viruses, the nucleocapsid is surrounded by a lipid bilayer derived from the modified host cell membrane and studded with an outer layer of virus envelope glycoproteins. They cause many diseases like common cold to AIDS, Covid-19.

Structure of Virus

- A basic structure of virus is nucleic acid core (either DNA or RNA but not both) surrounded by protein coat.
- Central core of nucleic acid of a virus is called genome and the protein coat surrounding is called as capsid.
- In some virus, an envelope made up of glycoprotein and phospholipid bilayer is present outside the capsid.

The basic structural components of a virus are;

1. Genome:

Virus contains either DNA or RNA as genetic material but not both. Virus which contains DNA as genetic material are called DNA virus and those containing RNA are called RNA virus.

A viral genome may consist of linear or circular ds DNA, single stranded DNA, ss linear RNA or ds linear RNA. Examples; Reo virus is a RNA virus which contains ds RNA genome. Parvovirus contains ss DNA, Papovavirus contains ds circular DNA as genetic materials.

2. Capsid:

Capsid is the outer layer. Sometime it is referred as coat or shell. Capsid serves as impenetrable shell around the nucleic acid core. Capsid also helps to introduce viral genome into host cell during infection. The protein coat or capsid is made up of number of morphological similar sub units called capsomere. Each capsomere is further composed of protomere.

Capsomere are arranged tightly together in a repetitive pattern to form complete capsid. The complete complex of nucleic acid and protein coat of a virus particle is called as virus nucleo-capsid. Structure of capsid give the symmetry to the virus. Virus particle may be either cubicl or helical or binal or complex symmetry.

3. Envelope:

Some virus contains envelope that surrounds nucleocapsid. The virus without envelope is called naked virus. The envelope is a bilayer of lipoprotein and glycoprotein. In some virus the glycoprotein projects out in the form of spike called peplomere. Some of the peplomers or glycoprotein spike such as Haemaglutinin and Neuraminidase which are involved in binding of virus to host cell.

4. Enzymes:

Some virus contains enzymes which play central role during infection process. Eg., Some bacteriophage contains an enzyme lysozyme, which makes small hole in bacterial cell that allows viral nucleic acid to get in. Some virus contains their own nucleic acid polymerase which transcribe the viral genome into mRNA during replication process. Eg., Retro virus are RNA virus that replicates inside host cell as DNA intermediate. These viruses possess an RNA dependent DNA polymerase called reverse transcriptase.

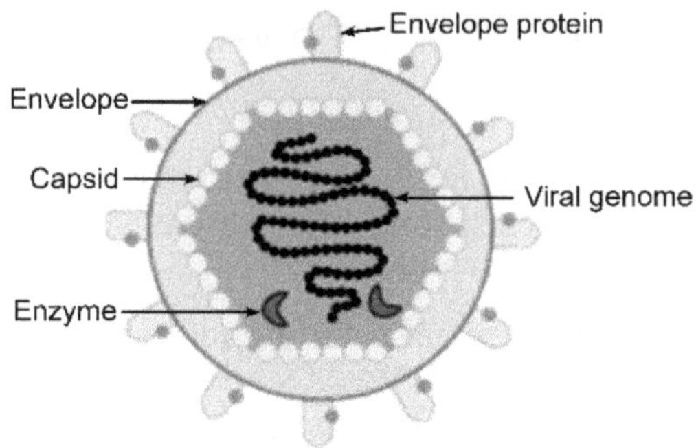

Depending upon the morphology of capsid, viruses can be classified into;

1. Helical Viruses
2. Polyhedral Viruses
3. Enveloped Viruses
4. Complex viruses

Helical Virus:

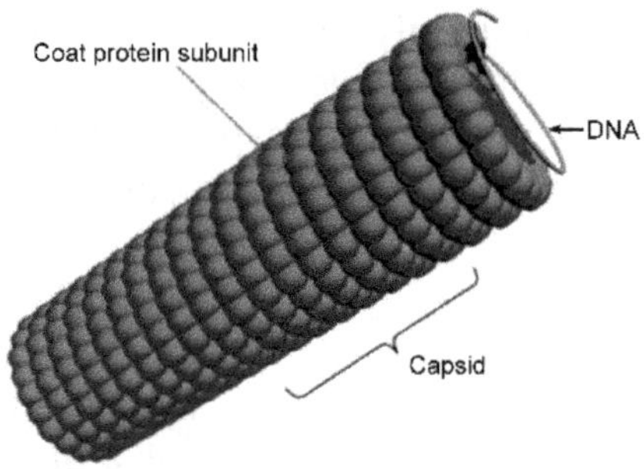

Helical viruses appear as rigid or flexible long rods. The nucleic acid is present within cylindrical capsid. The length of the virus is dependent on the length of the nucleic material. Single unit of the capsid is called a capsomer. E.g. Rabies Virus, Tobacco mosaic virus.

Polyhedral Viruses:

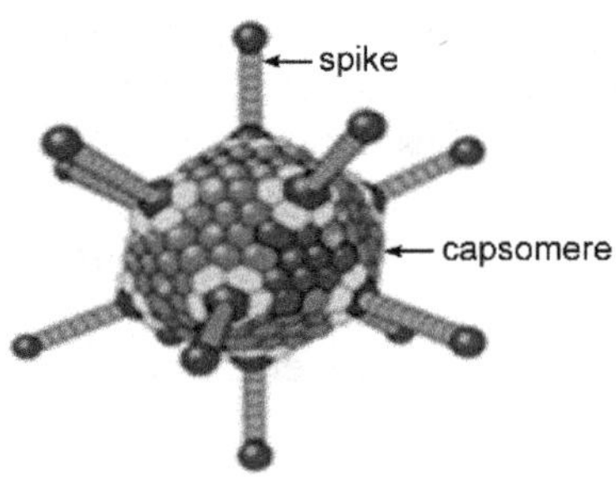

polyhedral virus

They are also called "Icosahedral" viruses. The regular polyhedron contains around 20 triangular faces and 12 corners. The nucleic acid along with certain proteins is stored in the core. E.g. Polio virus.

Enveloped Viruses:

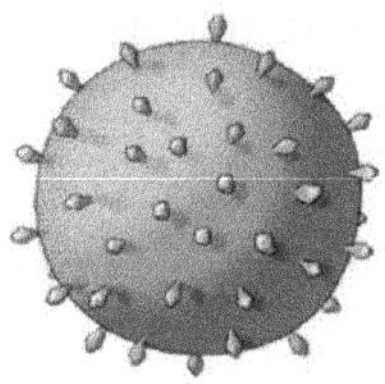

Roughly spherical and highly pleomorphic (Change in shape). Polyhedral or helical virus after enclosing in an envelope becomes enveloped viruses. The envelope of viruses provides protection and impart infectivity to them. Eg. Influenza virus, Herpes simplex virus.

Complex Viruses:

Structure of bacteriophage

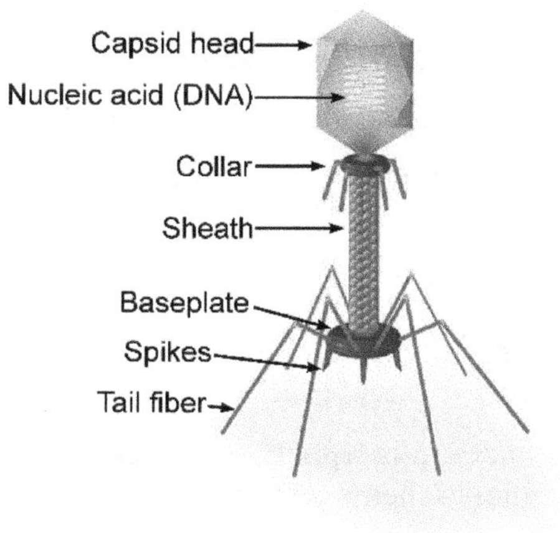

Some bacteriophages possess characteristic structure hence referred to as complex viruses. Their nucleic acid is packed in a hexagonal head, which is attached to a terminal tail. Tail may be surrounded with a contractile sheath. The terminal end of the tail has a basal plate. The basal plate has attached six pins and six tail fibers that help in binding to the specific receptor on the bacterial cell.

Classification

Depending upon the host in which they infect, viruses can be divided into three categories;

Bacterial Viruses contain DNA infect bacteria (Phaginea), Plant virus contain RNA infect plants (Phytophaginea), Animal viruses contain either DNA/ RNA infect humans and animals (Zoophagineae).

Depending upon the presence of genetic material, viruses can be divided into three categories;

DNA viruses: DNA is the genetic material e.g. parvovirus, papillomavirus, and herpesvirus.

RNA viruses: RNA is the genetic material e.g. Rotavirus, polio virus, yellow fever virus, dengue virus, hepatitis C virus, measles virus, rabies virus, influenza virus and Ebola virus, etc.

DNA-RNA viruses: In exceptional cases contain both DNA & RNA. Eg. RNA tumour viruses are called Leukoviruses and Rous's viruses.

Depending upon the mode of transmission, viruses can be divided into five categories;

Virus transmitted through respiratory route: Eg, Swine flu, Rhinovirus

Virus transmitted through faeco-oral route: Eg. Hepatitis A virus, Polio virus, Rota virus

Virus transmitted by sexual contacts: Eg. Retrovirus

Virus transmitted through blood transfusion: Eg. Hepatitis B virus, HIV

Zoonotic virus: Virus transmitted by biting of infected animals; Eg. Rabies virus, Alpha virus, Flavivirus

Baltimore Classification

The most commonly used system of virus classification was developed by Nobel Prize-winning biologist David Baltimore in the early 1970s.

In addition to the differences in morphology and genetics mentioned above, the Baltimore classification scheme groups viruses according to how the mRNA is produced during the replicative cycle of the virus.

Group I: viruses contain double-stranded DNA (dsDNA) as their genome. Their mRNA is produced by transcription in the same way as that of cellular DNA.

Group II: viruses have single-stranded DNA (ssDNA) as their genome. They convert their single-stranded genomes into a dsDNA intermediate before transcription to mRNA.

Group III: viruses have dsRNA as their genome. The strands separate, and one of them is used as a template for the generation of mRNA using the RNA-dependent RNA polymerase encoded by the virus.

Group IV: viruses have ssRNA as their genome with a positive polarity, which means that the genomic RNA can serve directly as mRNA.

Group V: viruses contain ssRNA genomes with a negative polarity, meaning that their sequence is complementary to the mRNA. The negative-stranded genome can be converted directly to mRNA.

Additionally, full-length positive RNA strands are made to serve as templates for the production of the negative-stranded genome.

Group VI: viruses have diploid (two copies) ssRNA genomes that must be converted, using the enzyme reverse transcriptase, to dsDNA; the dsDNA is then transported to the nucleus of the host cell and inserted into the host genome. Then, mRNA can be produced by transcription of the viral DNA that was integrated into the host genome.

Group VII: Viruses have partial dsDNA genomes and make ssRNA intermediates that act as mRNA, but are also converted back into dsDNA genomes by reverse transcriptase, necessary for genome replication.

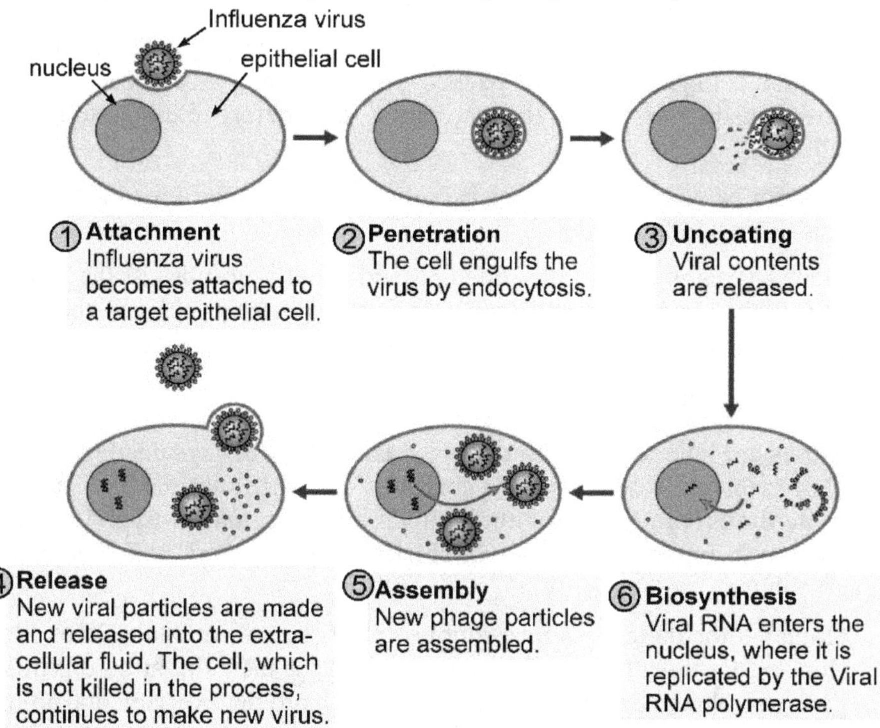

Fig 3.5. Mode of replication.

Steps of Replication of Virus

1. **Attachment:** Protein produced on the surface of the virus capsid or envelope binds to the specific receptor of the host cell surface. This binding process acts as a lock and key method where each key fits only with a specific lock.
2. **Penetration:** HIV and influenza virus with an envelope enters the cell with a fusion of host cell membrane whereas non-enveloped virus enters by translocation or through receptor mediated endocytosis. While penetrating, viral capsid protein goes into several conformation changes.
3. **Uncoating/disassembly:** The viral nucleic acid are released by the viral enzyme or host enzyme that degrades the viral capsid and uncoats the genetic material and makes it available for transcription and translation.
4. **Genome replication:** Transcription and translation are initiated after the uncoating of viral genetic material where DNA and RNA virus replicates in terms of different taxonomic grouping.
5. **Assembly:** After replication, the newly replicated genomic material are assembled together and are packed inside the new nucleocapsid of the virus. This process is also the maturation stage before release into the host cell.
6. **Release:** New viruses gets ready to be released in the host organism by lysis or by budding.

Enveloped virus is released by budding and usually do not kill the infected cell. So, they are termed as cytopathic virus. Whereas, lysis is termed as cytolytic which results in the death of the host cell.

Cultivation of Virus

As viruses are intracellular obligatory parasites, they always need living cells for their growth. They cannot be grown on any artificial media. There are **three methods** employed for the cultivation of animal viruses 1. Animal inoculation 2. Embryonated eggs or chick embryo method. 3. Tissue culture or cell culture.

1. Animal Inoculation – Susceptible experimental animals like Mice, Monkey, Rabbits, Guinea Pigs etc. are used for the cultivation of viruses. Virus sample to be cultivated should injected into the experimental animal. It is important to select specific host animal for particular viruses. Route of inoculation of viral sample in the host cell also play important role in cultivation of viruses. Other factors such as age and immunity of host animal also affect the growth of viruses in the host. Eg. Mice are the most widely employed animals in virology. It can be inoculated by routes like

intracerebral, subcutaneous, intraperitoneal or intranasal. The growth of the virus in inoculated animals may be indicated by death, disease or visible lesion. Disadvantages of animal inoculation are that immunity may interfere with viral growth.

2. Embryonate Eggs or Chick embryo method Good pasture (1931) was the first who used hen's embryonated egg for the cultivation of viruses. Embryonated egg provides several sites for the cultivation of viruses. Viz 1. Chorio- allantoic membrane 2. Allantoic cavity 3. Amniotic cavity 4. Yolk sac 5. Embryo Different site is used for growth of different viruses. Eg. Chorio-allantoic membrane is used for the cultivation of pox virus. Allantoic cavity is employed for the Influenza virus. There are several advantages, chick embryos are packed in their shells and have natural resistant against bacterial contamination. Chick embryo method is cheaper and easy to handle.

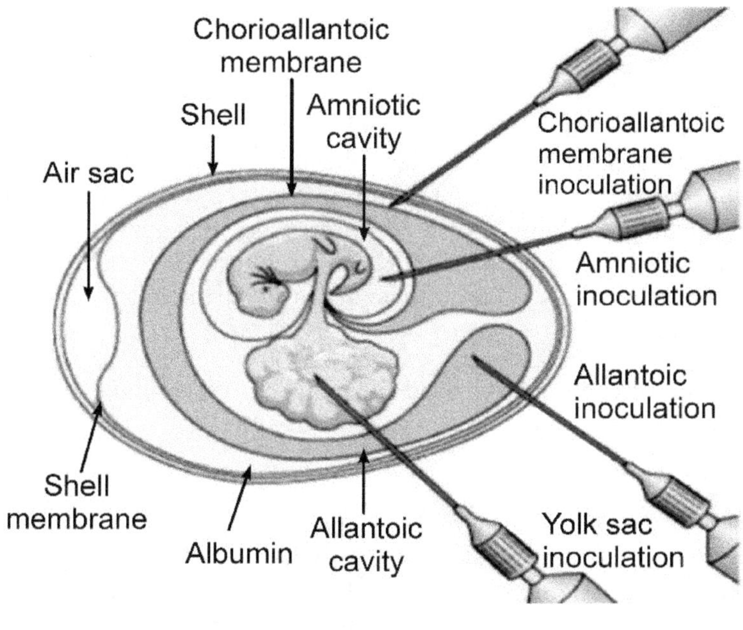

Fig 3.6. Chick embryo method.

3. Tissue Culture

Tissue Culture Steinhardt and colleagues (1913), was the first who used bits of tissue or organ for the cultivation of viruses. Now advance techniques are develop in Tissue culture. Three types of tissue cultures are available. 1. Organ culture:- Small bits of organs are used for the cultivation of virus. 2. Explants culture:- Fragments of minced tissue can be grown as 'explants' embedded in plasma clots.

3. Cell culture: - This is most common method for viral cultivation and growth of viruses.

Different types of cell cultures are used for different viruses. General method is as follows:

1. Tissue like Monkey Kidney, Rabbit Kidney is taken and treated with proteolytic enzymes such as Trypsin and by mechanical shaking, tissues are dissociated into the component cells. Trypsin, the protecolytic enzyme digest the binding material that binds the cells together in a tissue and results into free cells. He La cells (i.e. human cells from cervical cancer region) are also commonly used cell system for the cultivation of viruses.
2. After treatment with trypsin, cells are washed, counted and suspended in the growth medium.
3. Growth medium constitutes all those essential elements required for the growth of cell viz. essential amino acids, vitamins, salts, glucose, bicarbonates (buffer) with atmosphere containing 5% CO2 and supplemented with 5% calf serum.
4. Antibiotics are added into the growth medium to prevent bacterial contaminants. Some indicators like phenol red, neutral red etc. are added into the growth medium, change in indicator colour in growth medium, indicates the growth of virus in cell culture. In such growth medium cells divides and multiply. Then these cells are dispensed in bottle or petri plates. On incubation, cells divide to form a confluent monolayer sheet of cells occur within a week.

Various types of cell cultures used for virus cultivation are –

1. Primary cell culture
2. Diploid cell strains
3. Continuous cell lines.

1. **Primary cell culture: -** Derived form normal cells (eg. Monkey kidney tissue). The fresh monolayer of the cell is referred as Primary culture. They are capable of only limited growth in culture and cannot maintained in serial culture. Primary cell cultures are used during cultivation of viruses for vaccine production.
2. **Diploid cell strains: -** These are cells of a single type that retain the original diploid chromosome number and karyotype (appearance of two sets of chromosomes) during serial sub cultivation for a limited number of times. They are also employed for the production of viral vaccine.
3. **Continuous cell lines: -** These are the cells of single type, usually derived from cancer cells, that are capable of continuous serial cultivation indefinitely. Eg. Human cancer cells Viz. He La, Hep – 2 and KB lines

have been used for many years. These cell lines are stored in the cold (-700c) for use when necessary. The karyotype of these cells is aneuploid (a variable multiple of the haploid chromosome number.) Continuous cell lines are now widely useful in cultivating many types of viruses.

DETECTION OF VIRAL GROWTH

Viral growth in cell culture can be detected by the following methods

a. **Cytopathic effect (CPE)** Due to the viral growth, morphology of cultured cell change, these changes can be readily observed under microscope. These morphological changers in cell culture is called Cytopathic effect (CPE) and viruses causing CPE are called cytopathogenic virus. Eg. Adeno virus cause large granular clumps in cell culture.

b. **Fluorescence Antibody Technique (FAT): -** In this technique, cell from virus infected cultures can be stained by fluorescent conjugated antigen. Fluorescent dye such as fluorescein isothioacynate and rhodamine are generally used to tag with antibodies. FAT is very useful in testing for rabies virus in clinical specimen within few hours with 100% accuracy.

c. **Haemagglutination: -** Haemagglutination is the phenomenon of clumping of RBCs. Viruses such as mumps, measles and influenza can able to agglutinate the RBCs. their presence can be indicated by addition of guinea pig erythrocytes to the culture. If the viruses are cultivated in the cell culture, the erythrocytes will adsorb onto the cell surface also called 'haemadsorption.'

Disinfection is a process of removal or destruction of microorganisms and reducing their number to a non-harmful level. Disinfection usually kills the vegetative form of microorganisms and doesn't affect the endospores. The chemical which is used for disinfection of the non-living objects (Inanimate objects) is called a "Disinfectant".

The chemical which is used for disinfection of the living objects is called an "Antiseptic".

Mostly the disinfectants are "Bactericidal" while some may be "Bacteriostatic".

Ideal properties of Disinfectants:

Economical, Easy to use, Non-toxic, Broad Spectrum, Compatible with surface in use, odourless, Fast action, Good solubility / miscibility, No impact of physical factors, Good stability.

Classification of Disinfectants:

1) Acids and Alkalis 2) Alcohols 3) Aldehydes 4) Detergents and Soaps 5) Dyes 6) Halogens 7) Heavy Metals 8) Phenol and derivatives 9) Quaternary Ammonium Compounds.

Acids and Alkalis:

Acids produce their germicidal action by producing **H^+ ions**. e.g. Benzoic acid, Salicylic acid etc.

Alkalies produce their germicidal action by generating "**OH^- ions**". Only weak acids and alkalis are used as disinfectant as strong acids and alkalis are corrosive in nature.

Alcohols:

Alcohols exhibit rapid bactericidal action. They act by denaturation of microbial proteins and causing dehydration. Alcohols are also known to damage lipid blocks present in microbial cell membranes. Ethyl Alcohol (60-70%) is the most commonly used disinfectant among alcohols. Isopropanol is used in lower concentration that Ethanol i.e. 50-60% v/v.

Higher alcohols (Butyl Alcohol, Isopropyl Alcohol, Amyl Alcohol) are stronger in disinfectant action than ethyl alcohol. Alcohols are commonly used to disinfect the skin prior to the hypodermic injections. Alcohols above 60% concentration are found useful against viruses.

Aldehydes: Formaldehyde and Glutaraldehyde are commonly used aldehydes for disinfection. Formaldehyde is used in both gaseous as well as in liquid state. Formaldehyde is assumed to form cross linking with amino acids present on cell membrane and protein precipitation. Formaldehyde has a pungent odour and causes irritation to the eyes. Glutaraldehyde is less toxic and less irritant and possesses rapid sporicidal and tuberculocidal actions.

Detergents and Soaps:

These are widely used as **Surface active agents**, **wetting agents** and as **emulsifiers**. They are sub categorized in to following categories,

Anionic Surfactants. e.g. **Soaps**, Sodium Lauryl Sulphate.

Cationic Surfactants. e.g. **Cetrimide**, Benzalkonium chloride.

Amphoteric surfactants. e.g **Tego Compounds**.

Cationic Surfactant are the most effective disinfectant of this class. They bond with lipids present in cell wall and result in lysis of cell. Soaps prepared from saturated fatty acids are effective against Gram negative bacteria. While soaps prepared from unsaturated fatty acids are effective against Gram positive bacteria.

Dyes:

Basic dyes are more effective than acidic dyes. They act by inhibiting cellular oxidation process. Triphenyl methane and Acridine dyes are potent members of this class. Acridine dyes e.g. Proflavine, Aminacrine, Enflavine etc. act by demolishing DNA complexes of microbes and commonly used in treatment of burns and in ophthalmic applications and bladder irrigation. Triphenylmethane dyes e.g Crystal violet, Brilliant green, Malachite green act by inhibiting microbial cellular oxidation process.

Halogens:

Chlorine, Fluorine, Bromine and Iodine have strong antibacterial action. Fluorine, Bromine are well known irritants and hence not used as disinfectants. Iodine is comparatively safer. Chlorine is specially used for disinfection of water; its germicidal action is due to formation of Hypochlorous acid when it reacts with water. Chlorine acts by combining with cellular proteins and bacterial enzymes making them ineffective. Iodine is sporicidal, fungicidal and virucidal. Iodine is a strong oxidizing agent and causes inactivation of microbial proteins. Iodine is combined with surfactants like (Polyvinyl Pyrrolidone) to form compounds called "Iodophors". Iodophors are non-irritant, non-staining and odourless compounds.

Heavy Metal:

Mercury, Silver and copper compounds are common heavy metals. They act by combining with microbial proteins causing denaturation. The common compounds used are,

Mercury: Concentration (1:100 / 1:1000)

Mercuric chloride, Mercuric oxide., Metaphen.

Silver: Concentration (1:1000)

Silver Nitrate, Organic Colloidal Silver: Argyrol, Collargol.

Copper:

Copper Sulphate, (**Fungicide**, prevents algae growth in swimming pools.)

Phenol and derivatives:

Used by Lister in 1867 for first antiseptic surgery. It is obtained by distillation of coal tar. It has strong antimicrobial action and is used as a standard in evaluation of the efficiency of other disinfectants. They cause precipitation of cellular proteins and inactivation of bacterial enzymes. Cresol becomes more potent than phenol when mixed with soap, popular brand Lysol is nothing but a cresol in a soap solution.

Quaternary Ammonium Compounds:

Most Cationic Surfactants are Quaternary Ammonium Compounds. Their Action is by disruption of cell wall and membrane, inactivation of cellular proteins. They are effective against bacteria, fungi and certain protozoa.

Factors affecting disinfection, antiseptics and their evaluation.

Disinfection is a process of removal or destruction of microorganisms and reducing their number to a non-harmful level. Disinfection usually kills the vegetative form of microorganisms and doesn't affect the endospores.

The chemical which is used for disinfection of the non-living objects (Inanimate objects) is called a "Disinfectant". The chemical which is used for disinfection of the living objects is called an "Antiseptic".

Mostly the disinfectants are "Bactericidal" while some may be "Bacteriostatic".

Factors affecting action of Disinfectants:

The rate and extent of antibacterial action of the disinfectant depends on many factors like,

1) Concentration of the disinfectant 2) Chemical Structure of the disinfectant 3) Formulation of the disinfectant 4) Interfering substances in the environment 5) pH of the surrounding 6) Potentiation and antagonism of the disinfectants 7) Surface Tension 8) Temperature 9) Time of Contact 10) Type and no. of microbe's present.

1. Concentration of the disinfectant:

The rate of killing the microbes varies directly with concentration of the disinfectant. The rate of killing is related exponentially with the concentration of the disinfectant, not linearly. There is an optimum concentration of the disinfectant at which it shows maximum efficacy, below and beyond this concentration the efficacy decreases.

The Dilution Coefficient is an important characteristic of a disinfectant which determines how much dilution is to be made for maximum efficiency. The dilution coefficient is calculated using following formula,

$$n = \frac{logt2 - logt1}{logc1 - logc2}$$

Where, n=Dilution Coefficient of the Disinfectant, t1= Death time @ Concentration C1, t2= Death time @ Concentration C2.

2. Chemical Structure of the disinfectant:

Chemical activity is largely dependent on the chemical structure of the disinfectant. Introduction of an alkyl chain at para position of Phenol increases the activity, however, when the chain increases more than 6 carbon atoms it decreases the solubility and disinfectant action. Halogenation increases antimicrobial action of the phenol while nitration reduces it.

3. Formulation of the disinfectant:

A good formulation increases the effectiveness of the disinfectant. Iodine is virtually insoluble in water and hence is made to dissolve by using alcohol and potassium iodide solution. Addition of a surfactant in iodine solution decreases its odour, staining problem and increases stability of the preparation. Chlorhexidine and Quaternary ammonium compounds show increased efficiency in 70% alcohol solution than in the aqueous solution.

4. Interfering substances in the environment:

The organic materials like pus, blood etc present at site of action of disinfectant greatly reduces the activity of disinfectant. Presence of fats and oils at the site of action of phenol greatly reduces its activity.

5. pH of the surrounding:

Most bacteria show optimum growth at 6-8 pH. Acidic disinfectant shows maximum activity at an acidic pH as they remain ionized. Basic dyes like Acridine and Quaternary ammonium compounds show maximum activity at basic pH as they remain ionized at that pH. Amphoteric surfactants e.g. Tego compounds show good activity at variety of pH.

6. Potentiation and antagonism of the disinfectants:

Some disinfectants potentiate the activity of other disinfectants while some antagonize actions of each other. Potentiation: enhanced antimicrobial activity by addition of any excipients. Eg., Polysorbate80 addition with disinfectants.

Synergism: enhanced antimicrobial activity by addition of two antimicrobial or disinfectants Eg., Different esters of p-hydroxybenzoate are available, when combined together exhibit synergistic activity

Antagonism: Decreased antimicrobial activity by addition of any excipients Eg., Sodium thiosulphate, lubrol, lecithin etc.

7. Surface Tension:

Surface tension is the tendency of liquid surfaces to shrink into the minimum surface area possible.

The lowered surface tension in an aqueous solution of the disinfectant increases its adsorption on the microbial cell and increases wetting properties and solubility of the solution. A combination of Phenol with soap shows increased disinfectant action as soap by its property lowers surface tension.

8. Temperature:

The action of disinfectant normally increases with temperature at a certain point above which it decreases. The effect of temperature on disinfectant action is expressed by using "Temperature coefficient" which is denoted by "***θ***", whereas per 10°C is denoted by Q10.

The Q10 is calculated using following formula,

$$Q10 = \frac{TimeRequiredtokillatT}{TimeRequiredtokillat(T+10)}$$

9. Time of Contact:

Sufficient time of contact must be allowed to the disinfectant to show its action. The lesser time of contact results in decreased activity of the disinfectant.

10.Type and no. of microbe's present:

Disinfectants are mainly active against vegetative forms of microbes and not their spore form. Bacterial spores are very difficult to destroy however, aldehydes like formaldehyde are known sporicidals. Acid fast bacilli due to presence of fats in their cell membrane are virtually immune to aqueous solutions of disinfectants but can be killed using phenols, aldehydes and halogen derivatives.

EVALUATION OF DISINFECTANTS

Mostly the disinfectants are "Bactericidal" while some may be "Bacteriostatic". Minimal inhibitory concentration (MIC) is the lowest concentration of a chemical agent or drug that inhibits growth of a particular microorganism. The MIC is not a constant for a given chemical agent because it is affected by many factors like, nature of the target microorganism, inoculum size, composition of the culture medium, incubation time, conditions of incubation such as temperature, pH and aeration.

The common methods used for evaluation of a disinfectant are as follows,

1)Tube Dilution Method 2) Agar Plate Method 3) Filter Paper & Cup Plate Method, 4) Ditch-Plate Method 5) Phenol Coefficient Method 6) Kelsey Sykes Method.

1. Tube Dilution Method:

In this method, a series of tubes is set up, each containing the same quantity of a standard growth liquid medium (Commonly Mueller-Hinton broth) and a gradually increasing concentration of the disinfectant to be tested. The tubes are then inoculated with the same quantity of cell suspension of the test microorganism and incubated for 2-3 days @ 30-35°C.

The first tube in the series where there is complete absence of growth of the test microorganism denotes the minimal inhibitory concentration (MIC) of the disinfectant.

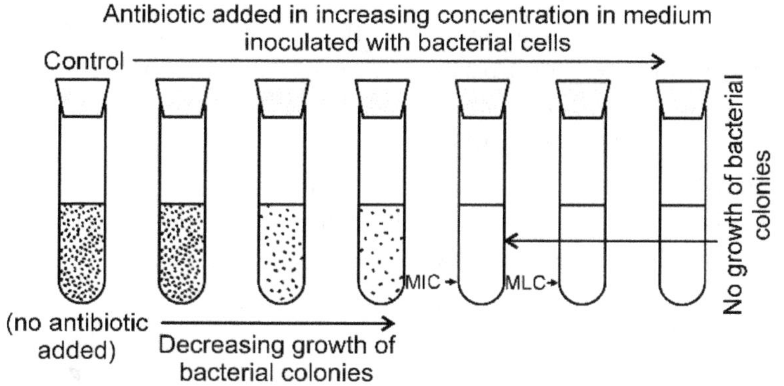

Fig 3.7. Tube dilution method.

2. Agar Plate Method:

It is very similar to the tube dilution method. In this method, Petri plates containing a standard growth agar medium (usually Mueller-Hinton agar) are taken at the place of lubes containing liquid medium. Disinfectants of various concentrations are inoculated on the agar surface of plates already inoculated with the same quantity of the test microorganism. Plates are incubated and then examined for growth. The first plate in the series where there is complete absence of growth of the test microorganism denotes the minimal inhibitory concentration (MIC) of the disinfectant.

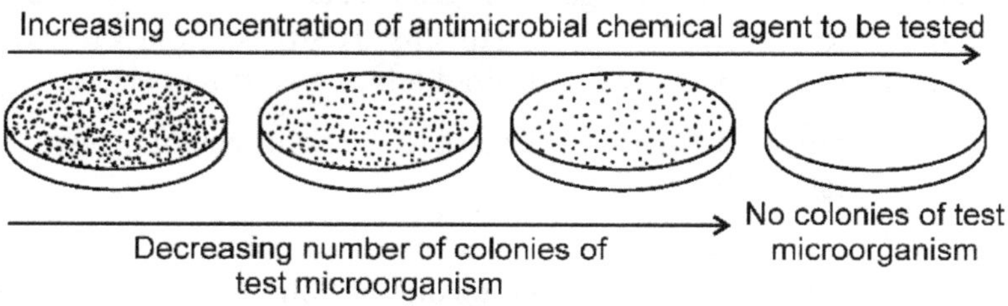

Fig 3.8. Agar plate method.

3. Filter Paper & Cup Plate Method:

These methods are known as "Agar Diffusion Tests". The agar is melted and cooled @ 45°C, inoculated with test microorganisms and poured in a sterile petri plate.

In case of "Cup Plate Method" when the agar is solidified the holes of 9 mm diameter were made by using sterile corn borer and the disinfectant is directly placed in it.

In case of the Filter Paper method the filter paper disks soaked in disinfectant solution are placed in the holes.

The zone of inhibition is observed after incubation @ 30-35 °C. During incubation, the disinfectant diffuses into the agar. The diameter of the zone of inhibition gives indication of activity of the disinfectant, larger the diameter greater is the efficiency of the disinfectant.

A zone of Inhibition is proportional to the amount of the antimicrobial agent added to the filter paper disc, the solubility of the agent, the diffusion coefficient, and the overall effectiveness of the agent.

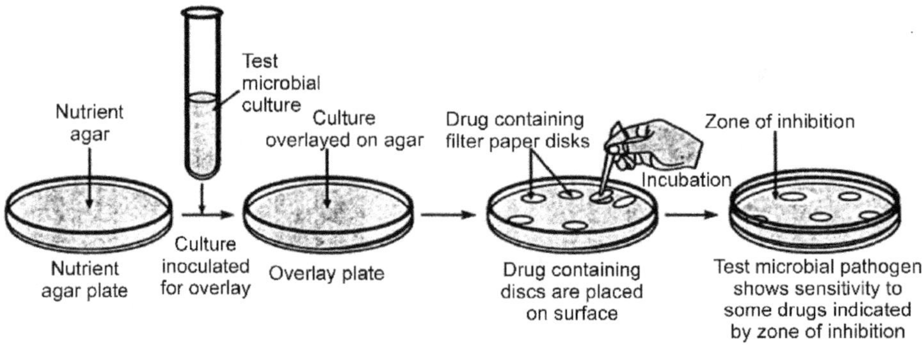

Fig. 3.9. Filter Paper & Cup Plate Method.

4. Ditch-Plate Method:

Agar is melted and then solidified in a petri plate. A ditch is made in the petri plate by cutting the soliodified agar. The disinfectant solution is made to run through the ditch carefully. The test organisms are streaked outwards from the ditch. The petriplate is incubated at desired temp. And time period.

The microorganisms which are resistant to the disinfectant grow even near the start at the ditch itself.

The sensitive organisms show a zone of inhibition near the ditch or at center of the petri plate. The width of the zone of inhibition is an indication of activity against the test organism.

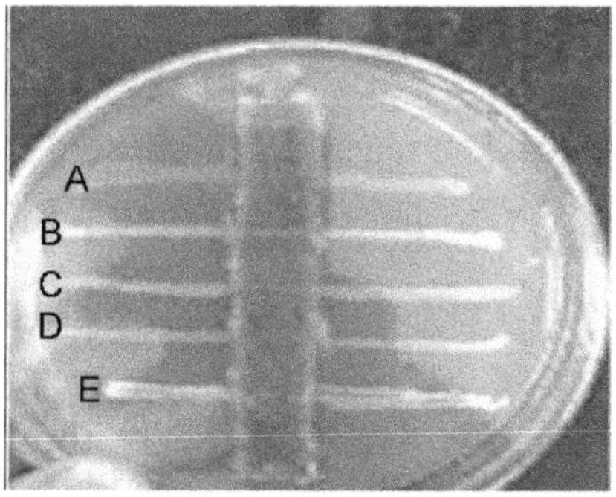

Fig. 3.10. Ditch plate method.

5. Phenol Coefficient Method:

In this method the efficacy of the disinfectant in use is rated by comparing it with the activity of Phenol taking as a standard. The test is carried out by adding an increasing amount of phenol and disinfectant in test tubes containing microorganisms.

In UK the test organism used is Salmonella typhi while the USA uses Salmonella typhi, Staphylococcus aureus and Pseudomonas aeruginosa.

The official phenol coefficient tests include

Rideal-Walker Test (RW Test), Chick-Martin Test, United States FDA Test for Phenol Coefficient. (FDA Test)

Rideal-Walker Test:

Introduced by Rideal and Walker the British chemists in 1903 are still in use. The test uses Rideal, Walker Broth and Salmonella typhi as a test organism. Different dilutions of the phenol and test disinfectants are made and 5 ml of each is inoculated with the 0.5 ml of the 24-hr broth culture of the test icroorganism.

All the test tubes are placed in a water bath at 17.5 °C. Subcultures from each test tube are taken and transferred to 5 ml sterile broth after 2.5, 5, 7.5 and 10 minutes. The broth tubes are incubated at 37 °C for 2 - 3 days and are examined for the presence or absence of the growth and the Phenol coefficient is calculated using the formula,

$$RW Coefficient = \frac{Dilution of Disinfectant Killing In 7.5 But Not In 5 min}{Dilution of Phenol Killing In 7.5 But Not In 5 min}$$

The Phenol Coefficient for phenol is considered as "1" any value for disinfectant coming below one is considered as less while above it is more.

Advantages of Phenol Coefficient Test:

Quick, Inexpensive, Reproducible results, Useful to eliminate useless products, Sets standard for the preparations.

Disadvantages of Phenol Coefficient Test:

Most tests use only one test organism i.e. Salmonella typhi which represents inadequate information.

Compares the activity of disinfectants at only one concentration at fixed conditions. Presence of organic matter at action time is not considered.Does not give information about tissue toxicity of the disinfectant. Sampling errors are large.

6. Kelsey-Skyes Mehod:

Developed in 1969, this test overcomes many drawbacks of the RW Test.The test uses several test organisms viz. Staphylococcus aureus, Proteus vulgaris, Eschericia coli and Pseudomonas aeruginosa.

Tests can be carried out in a clean as well as dirty environment. In both clean and dirty cases, the final bacterial concentration should be about 10^9/ml.Clean conditions are simulated by using a clean broth while dirty conditions are simulated by using a yeast suspension or inactivated horse serum.

The samples are taken at 8, 18 and 28 minutes are then incubated at 30 to 32°C and observations of growth of microorganisms in test tubes are recorded.

Result interpretation: A disinfectant is considered satisfactory if, no growth in 2 or 5 tubes of 18 min sample or, no more than 5 colonies from 5 drops on the agar plate.

Sterility test

Sterilization is the process of complete removal of microorganisms from any surface or product. Sterility hence can be defined as "Complete freedom from microorganisms". A sterility test may be defined as - 'a test that critically assesses whether a sterilized pharmaceutical product is free from contaminating microorganisms. According to Indian Pharmacopoea (1996) the sterility testings are intended for detecting the presence of viable forms of microorganisms in or on the pharmacopoeal preparations.

The products which are to be strictly supervised for absence of the microorganisms are those who come directly in contact with the systemic circulation e.g. ophthalmic preparations, parenteral injections, implants, bandages, surgical dressings, needles, surgical instruments etc.

TEST FOR STERILITY: PHARMACEUTICAL PRODUCTS

Sterility tests can be carried out using one of the following methods,

Methods A: Membrane Filtration. Method B: Direct Inoculation

Method A: Membrane Filtration.

This method is preferred when substance to be tested is,

a) an oil, b) an ointment that can be put into solution, c) a non-bacteriostatic solid not readily soluble in the culture medium and d) a soluble powder or a liquid that possesses inherent bacteriostatic and fungistatic properties. For liquid products where the volume > 100ml or more.

Precautions:

A laminar sterile airflow cabinet – to avoid accidental contamination. Working conditions monitored regularly by sampling the air and surfaces of the working area.

Apparatus:

A suitable unit consists of a closed reservoir and a receptacle between which a properly supported membrane of appropriate porosity is placed. Nominal pore size not > 0.45µm and diameter of approx. 47mm.Flow rate is adjusted to 55-75 ml of water / minute. Pressure 70 mm of Hg. Cellulose nitrate filter for aqueous, oily and weakly alcoholic solutions. Cellulose acetate solution for strong alcoholic solutions.

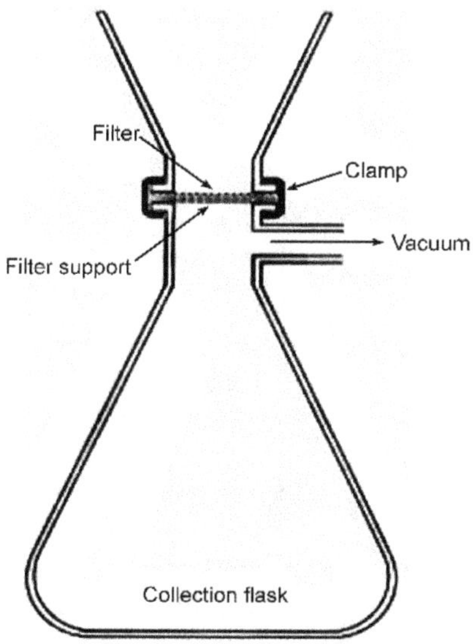

Fig. 3.11. Membrane Filtration method.

Dilution Fluids:

Fluid A: Dissolve 1g of peptic digest of animal tissue in water to make 1 liter, filter / centrifuge, adjust to pH 7.1±0.2, dispense into flasks in 100-ml quantities and sterilise at 121° for 20 minutes.

Fluid B: If the test sample contains lecithin or oil, **use fluid A** to **each liter of which has been added 1 ml of polysorbate 80,** adjust to pH 7.1±0.2, dispense into flasks in 100-ml quantities and sterilise at 121° for 20 minutes.

Quantities of sample to be used:

Quantities of sample to be used:

Preparation	Quantity in each container of the preparation	Minimum quantity to be used for each culture medium
Liquids	Less than 1 ml.	Total contents of container.
	1-40 ml	Half of the container but not less than 1 ml.
	40 ml to 100 ml.	20 ml
	More than 100 ml	10% of the container but not less than 20 ml.
Antibiotic liquids		1 ml
Other soluble preparations		The whole contents of each container to provide not less than 200mg.
Insoluble preparations ointments & creams.		The whole contents of each container to provide not less than 200mg.
Solids	Less than 50mg	Total container.
	50 mg - 300 mg	Half of the container but not less than 50 mg.
	300 mg - 5g	150 mg
	More than 5 gm	500 mg

Table contd...

Catgut and other surgical sutures for veterinary use.		Three sections of a strand each 30 cm long
Surgical dressings/ cotton/ gauze (In packages)		100 mg per package
Sutures and other individually packed single use material.		Whole device
Other medical devices		Whole device or material cut into pieces or diassembled

Method of test:

1. For aqueous solution: -

Prepare each membrane by aseptically transferring fluid A + media + preparation being examined.

Alternatively, first, combined quantities of preparation + prescribed in the two media. Draw the liquid rapidly through a filter with aid of vacuum. If the solution being examined has antimicrobial properties, wash the membrane by filtering 100ml of sterile fluid A, three times, or quantities should be sufficient to allow growth of small inoculum of organisms. After filtration, aseptically remove membrane from holder, cut the membrane in half, immerse one half of membrane in 100ml of soyabean-casein digest medium and incubate at 20° to 25° for not < 7days. Similar, other membranes in FTM (30° to 35°).

2. For liquids immiscible with aqueous vehicles and suspensions: - Same as above but add sufficient quantity of fluid A to achieve rapid filtration. Sometimes use sterile enzyme preparations such as penicillinase or cellulase to aid in dissolving insoluble substances. If lecithin is there, use fluid B for diluting.

3. For oils and oily solutions: Low viscous, filter without dilution through dry membrane.Viscous oils – dilute as per needed using sterile diluent like isopropyl myristate – filter by applying pressure or suction gradually. Wash the membrane at least 3 times sterile fluid B (100 ml) or to heat not > than 45° and use warm solutions for washing membrane.

4. For ointments and creams: Dilute ointments in a fatty base and emulsions of the w/o type to give a fluid concentration of 1%w/v, by heating (if necessary), not > than 40° with a suitable sterile diluent.

5. For soluble solids: Dissolve substance in a suitable sterile solvent for each medium and carry out test described under aqueous solutions.

6. For sterile devices: Aseptically pass a sufficient volume of fluid B through each of not less than 20 devices so that not less than 100ml is recovered from each device. Collect fluids in sterile containers and filter the entire volume through a membrane filter funnel, and follow the test as under for aqueous solutions.

Merits of Filtration Technique

Wide application – can be used for solutions, soluble solid, insoluble solids, oils, ointments, syringes like articles. Very large volume can be tested with one pad. Small volume of broth is required than direct inoculation into culture media. Apply to substances for which no satisfactory inactivators are known.

Some strong antibacterial agents like mercurial and quaternary ammonium compounds, inactivated by treatment with appropriate neutralising solution. Subculturing is often eliminated.

Demerits of Filtration Technique

The possibility of adsorption of sufficient medicament. Highly skilled staff and exceptionally good aseptic techniques are necessary. A virtually sterile environment is essential.

A room with laminar air flow and conventional asepsis laboratory is needed.

Method B Direct Inoculation

Method of test:

1. For aqueous solutions and suspensions:

Remove liquid from test containers with a sterile pipette or with a sterile syringe or a needle. Aseptically transfer specified volume of the material from each container to a vessel of the culture medium. Mix the liquid with the medium but do not aerate excessively. Incubate the inoculated media for not less than 14 days, unless otherwise specified in the monograph. Incubate at 30° to 35°C in case of fluid thioglycolate medium and at 20° to 25°C in case of soyabean casein digest medium.

If a test sample renders the medium turbid, it is difficult to examine presence or absence of microbial growth by visual examination. Transfer suitable portions of the same medium to fresh vessels between the third and seventh days after the test is started. Continue incubation of transfer vessels for not less than 7 additional days after the transfer and for a total of not less than 14 days.

2. For oils and oily solutions: In media, add 0.1% w/v of (4 –tert - octylphenoxy) polyethoxy ethanol, 1% w/v of polysorbate 80 or other suitable emulsifying agent, in an appropriate conc. Oil containing cultures should be shaken gently each day.

3. For ointments: Preparation is diluted tenfold in a sterile diluent such as fluid B or any other aqueous vehicle capable of dispersing test material homogeneously throughout the fluid mixture. Mix 10ml of fluid mixture with 80 ml of the medium and proceed the same as aqueous solutions & suspension.

4. For solids: Mix, and incubate same as 1)

5. For sterile devices: - For articles of such size and shape as permit complete immersion in not more than 1000ml of culture medium test the intact article, using the appropriate media and incubate same as 1).

For transfusion or infusion assemblies or where the size of an item makes immersion impracticable, flush the lumen of each of 20 units with a sufficient quantity of fluid thioglycolate medium and soyabean casein medium to yield a recovery of not less than 15ml of each medium, and incubate with not less than 100 ml of each of two media.

Where the presence of the specimen being tested interferes with the test because of bacteriostatic action, rinse the article thoroughly with minimum amount of fluid A. Recover the rinsed fluid and test as described for sterile devices under method A.

Observation and Interpretation of Results.

At interval during incubation period, and at its conclusion, examine media for macroscopic evidence of microbial growth.

If no evidence of growth is found, the preparation being examined passes the test for sterility.

If evidence of microbial growth is found, reserve the containers, and it is demonstrated that it is not due to preparation, hence the tests for sterility are invalid and may be recommenced. Perform a retest using the same number of samples, volumes to be tested and the media

If no evidence of microbial growth is then found, the preparation being examined passes the test for sterility.

If microbial growth is found, isolate and identify the organisms.

If they are not readily distinguishable from those growing in the containers reserved in the first test, the preparation being examined fails the test for sterility.

If they are readily distinguishable from those growing in the containers reserved in the first test, perform a second retest using twice the number of samples.

If no evidence of microbial growth is found in the second retest, the preparation being examined passes the test for sterility.

If evidence of growth of any micro-organisms is found in second retest, the preparation being examined fails the test for sterility.

UNIT - IV

Contamination and Prevention of Microbes

4.1 ASEPTIC AREA

4.1.1 Introduction

Aseptic techniques are employed to provide protection to ophthalmic and parenteral products by preventing the entry of microbial and particulate contamination. Prevention of microbial contamination is also required to remove pyrogens and toxic bacterial products. The terminally sterilised products (product sealed in container and then sterilised) are prepared in clean areas: while products not terminally sterilised are prepared under aseptic conditions using sterile materials or are sterilised by filtration before being packed in sterile containers. Such aseptic products are formulated or prepared in an aseptic area, which is a room within a clean area designed, constructed, serviced, and used for controlling and preventing microbial contamination of the product.

Like sterile medicinal products, vaccines containing dead micro-organisms, microbial extracts,or inactivated viruses are also filled in aseptic areas; while live or attenuated vaccines are filledin separate areas.

The goal of any facility is to design such an aseptic or sterile environment which provides a controlled environment so that the entrance of viable (microbial) and non-viable (particles) contaminants can be minimised. A controlled environment prevents cross-contamination of Compounded Sterile Preparations (CSPs). To reduce the contamination-related risk, all compounding should be done within primary engineering controls, like a Laminar Airflow Hood (LAFH), also known as workbenches, Biological Safety Cabinet (BSC), or a Compounding Aseptic Isolator (CA).

4.1.2 Designing of Aseptic Area

The sterile production unit and the general manufacturing area within the hospital pharmacy or factory should be located separately. The sterile production unit should be buffered, i.e., unauthorised personnel should not gain access to this unit.

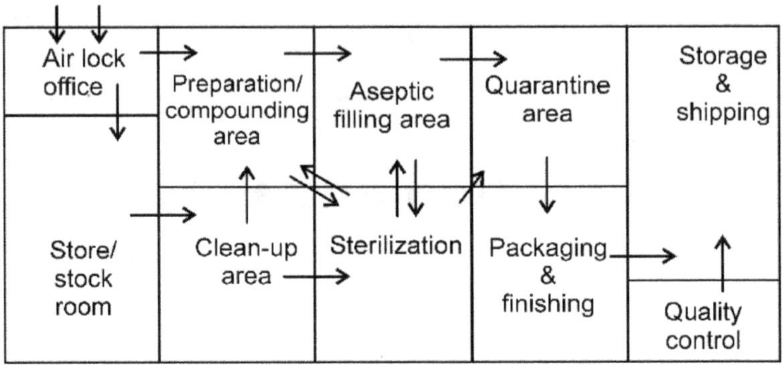

Fig.4.1 Flow Diagram of Aseptic Area.

The aseptic unit is designed to carry out each stage of production separately. The unit should also ensure a safe and organised workflow so that the need for personnel to move around the clean rooms is minimised. The unit is built and the equipment is positioned in such a manner that the product remains protected from contamination.

The layout of aseptic area should be such that cleaning can be done easily and dust accumulation can also be reduced. Arrangement should be such that the risk of cross- contamination (contamination of one product or material with another) is reduced.

The filling area should be adjacent to the compounding area where the personnel assemble andprepare materials utilised by the staff in the filling area. In figure 4.1 the layout of areas and rooms for preparing terminally sterilised products (such as small or large volume injections) isshown.

4.1.2.1 Design and Construction

Only authorised personnel can gain access to the clean and aseptic filling areas. The personnelenter the clean rooms by passing through the changing rooms where they put on and remove their clean room uniform.

A pass-Over (or cross-over) bench extends across the changing room to form a physical barrierfor separating the different areas for changing by the personnel.

Special precautions are taken for preventing clean and aseptic filling areas from getting contaminated while materials are being passed through airlocks or hatchways. Thus, sterilisersand entry ports are fitted with double-sided doors, which are interlocked to prevent simultaneous opening of both the doors.

4.1.2.2 Surfacing Materials

The floor, wall, and ceiling surface of clean rooms should be smooth, impervious, and unbroken to reduce the release and accumulation of contaminating particles and organisms. The surface material should be such that they can withstand the effects of cleaning agents anddisinfectants. The ceilings are scaled so that the contaminants do not enter from the space above them.

Uncleanable recesses should be avoided within the clean rooms to minimise the accumulation of contaminating particles. Thus, thc wall and floor junction should be covered. Minimum shelves, ledges, cupboards, and equipment should be present. Non-opening and sealed windows should be present to prevent the entry of contaminants.

4.1.2.3 Services

The piped liquids and gases entering the clean rooms should be filtered first, thus ensuring thatthe liquid or gas at the work position is as clean as the air in the clean room. The position of pipes and ducts should be such that they can be easily cleaned. Other fittings, like fuse boxes and switch panels should be placed outside the clean rooms.

Sinks and drains should not be present in areas where aseptic procedures are carried out withinthe clean room areas. They should nowhere be present in the complete unit. The areas having sinks and drains should be designed, positioned, and maintained such that the risk of microbialcontamination is reduced; therefore, they are fitted with easily cleanable traps, installed with electrically heated disinfection devices.

A limited number of doors and ports should be present for entry of personnel and materials, respectively. The entry doors should be self-closing to allow easy movement of the personnel.

Airlock doors, wall ports, through-the-wall autoclaves, and dry heat sterilisers should have interlocked doors to prevent simultaneous opening of both the doors. All the doors should havean alarm system which should ring when more than one door are being opened.

Lights in clean rooms should be fitted with the ceiling so that dust accumulation reduces and also the airflow pattern within the room is not disturbed. The equipment in clean rooms should be positioned such that accumulation of particles and microbial contaminants does not Occur.

4.1.3 Laminar Flow Equipment (Laminar Airflow Hood)

A Laminar Airflow Hood (LAFH)/ Laminar Aseptic Hoods, or a workbench, is a primary engineering control device which provides the following services during aseptic compounding

1. Clean air to the critical sites (immediate aseptic compounding area),
2. Constant flow of air out of the work area to prevent the entry of room air, and

3. Outward flow of air from the hood that suspends and removes contaminants which havebeen introduced in the work area by personnel.

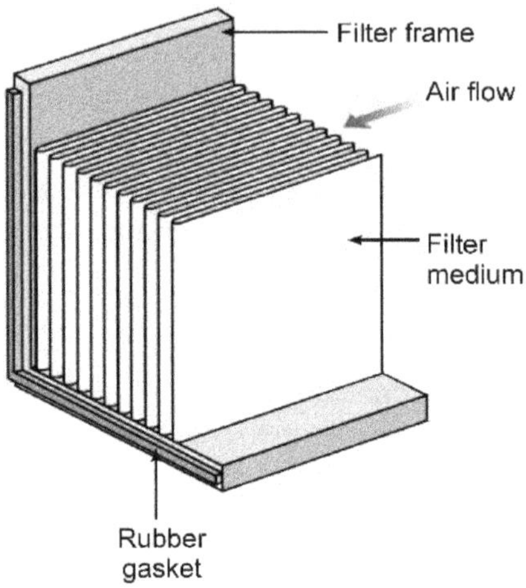

Fig.4.2 Section through a Mini-Pleat High-Efficiency Filter.

A High Efficiency Particulate Air (HEPA) Filter is the most important part of a LAFH. The airwithin the room is taken into this filter and passed through a pre-filter which removes the grosscontaminants (lint, dust, etc.). The air is then blown at a uniform velocity through the hood andHEPA filter in a unidirectional (laminar flow) manner over the critical sites (immediate asepticcompounding area). HEPA filter is a particulate filter which traps the airborne particles and microbes; but allows the gases to pass through.

HEPA filter should be fitted either at or near to the clean room inlet. A pre-filter is fitted upstream of the HEPA filter, thus extending the final filter's life. A fan is also fitted which pumps the air through the filter.

The filter medium used in HEPA filters 1S made up of pleated fiberglass paper. Parallelly arranged pleats not only increase the filter surface area but also the air flow through the filter (figure 10.2). This parallel arrangement of filter medium also allows the filter to retain a compact volume. In the traditional type of HEPA filters, aluminium foil was used as spacers, which are no longer used in the modern mini-pleat type of filter (now widely used). The mini- pleat filters have a shallower depth in construction than the traditional HEPA filter. The filter material is sealed to an aluminium frame within the filter (figure l0.2). One side of the filter isprotected with a coated mild steel mesh. HEPA filters provide:

1. A high air flow rate,
2. A high particulate holding capacity, and
3. A low-pressure drop across the filter.

HEPA filters remove larger, medium, and smaller particles from the air by inertial impaction, direct interception, and by Brownian diffusion, respectively. The HEPA filters are leas efficient in removing particles of about 0.3um size. However, its efficiency of removing particles is affected by air velocity and filter packing. It removes larger and smaller particles with more efficiency.

The LAFH works on the principle that twice-filtered laminar layers of aseptic air continuously sweep the work area within the hood to prevent the entry of contaminated room air.

4.1.3.1 Types

A laminar air flow hood is of two types:

1. **Horizontal Airflow Hoods:** These hoods (figure 10.3) sweep the filtered air from the backto the front of the hood. An electrical blower draws the contaminated room air using a pre-filter (similar to a furnace filter), to remove gross contaminants. The pre-filter demands timely cleanliness and replacement. The air after passing through the pre-filter is accelerated (but notpressurised) so that a consistent airflow distribution reaches the final filter (HEPA filter), present at the back portion of the hood's working area.

   HEPA filter removes 99.97% of 0.3μ or larger sized particles, thus removing most of the 0.5μor larger sized airborne microorganisms.

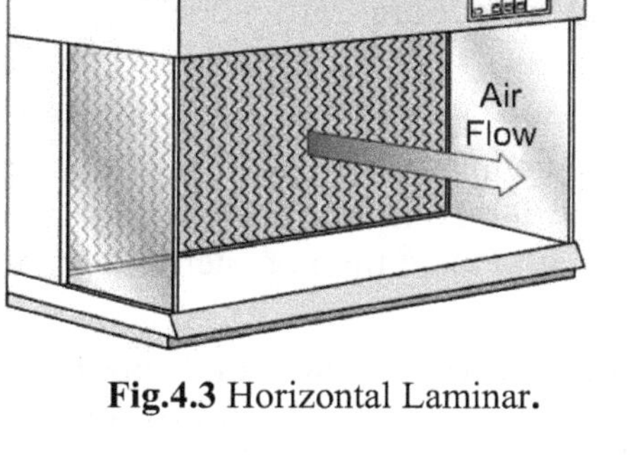

Fig.4.3 Horizontal Laminar.

2. **Vertical Airflow Hoods:** These hoods (figure 4.4) sweep the filtered air vertically. The airpassing through HEPA filter merges from the top and passes downward through the working area. The vertical airflow hoods work on the principle that the air flow between the HEPA filterand the component used for CSPs preparation should not be interrupted. When a

foreign object comes in between the sterile object and the HEPA filter, the wind turbulence (zone of turbulence) in the critical area increases, and foreign contaminants are carried to the sterile work surface, thus contaminating the injection port, needle, or syringe.

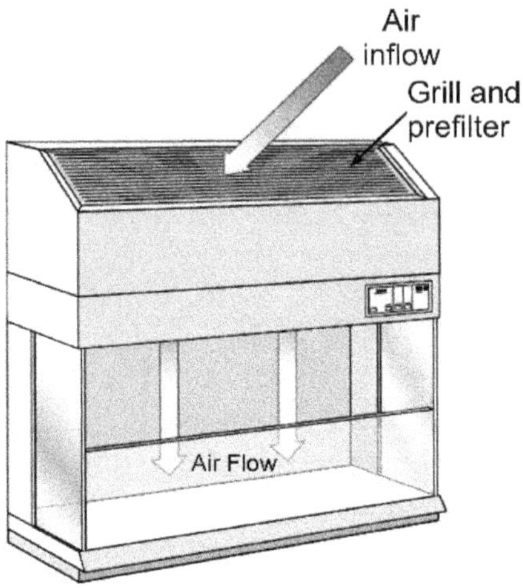

Fig.4.4 Vertical Laminar.

For ensuring complete sterility, nothing should pass behind a sterile object in a horizontal airflow hood; and in case of vertical airflow hood, nothing should pass above the sterile object. The materials within the compounding work area interrupt the pattern of air blowing from theHEPA filter.

4.1.3.2 Operating Principles

A Laminar Air Flow Hood (LAFH) operates on the following general principles:

1. It should be placed away from traffic, doors, air vents, or anything that can produce air currents, to avoid entrance of contaminants.
2. It should remain on for 24 hours otherwise, non-filtered, non-sterile air occupies the compounding work area. Thus, when again it is turned on, it should be left for 30 minutes for disinfection and then used. This also allows the hood to eliminate the non-sterile air from the compounding work area.
3. Before using the LAFH, its interior working surfaces should be disinfected using 70% isopropyl alcohol (or other suitable disinfecting agents) and a clean, lint-free cloth. Cleaning should be done efficiently beginning from the HEPA filter in a top-to-bottom and back-to-front motion, to completely remove the contaminants.
4. Cleaning should be done after every compounding batch and also when the work surface becomes dirty. Some materials on the surface are

insoluble in alcohol (e.g., dextrose and amino acids), thus sterile water is used initially. After wiping the water from the surface, it is then cleaned using alcohol. Plexiglas sides present in some types of LAFHs, should not be cleaned using alcohol but with warm water and a germicidal detergent (e.-g., Lysol IC, Vesphene, or LpH).

5. HEPA filter grill (protective grill) should be cleaned in such a way that it does not get wet.
6. Objects essential for aseptic compounding should be placed in the hood. Paper, pens, labels,or trays should not be placed in this area.
7. HEPA filter should not be brought into contact with cleaning solution, aspirate from syringes, and glass from ampoules (should not be opened towards the filter)
8. The operators during compounding should not wear any jewellery on hands or wrists since they affect the integrity of personnel clothing (gowns and gloves).
9. The operators should minimise talking and should cough away from the compounding workarea.
10. The operators should avoid or reduce the unnecessary movement within or around the LAFH to minimise the airflow turbulence.
11. Smoking, eating, gum chewing, and drinking are strictly prohibited in the aseptic environment.
12. The objects should be arranged to get full benefit of the laminar air flow. Critical items should be placed close to the air source. The objects in horizontal hood should not be placed closer than 3 inches from the back of the hood (ensuring that nothing should be in direct contactwith the filter). The pharmacist in some cases, may stack a few objects (such as IVPBs), but from lower to higher starting from the back of the hood. Also, the stack should contain only 3-4 objects.
13. The aseptic procedures should be carried out 6 inches away from the sides and front edge of the hood to prevent contamination.
14. Testing of primary engineering controls (e.g., LAFHs, BSCs, and CAIs) should be carriedevery 6 months by qualified personnel. Testing is also required whenever the device 1s moved, or the filter is damaged. Specific tests are used for the certification of integrity of airflow velocity and HEPA filter.

4.1.3.3 Uses

Given below are the uses of a laminar air flow hood:

1. It has various applications, especially where an individual clean air environment is required for smaller items, e.g., particle sensitive electronic devices.

2. It is used for special operations in laboratories.
3. It can be tailor made to the specific requirements of laboratories and are also used for general lab work, especially in medical, pharmaceutical, electronic, and industrial sectors.

4.1.3.4 Advantages

Given below are the advantages of a laminar air flow hood:

1. The sterile area is spacious.
2. Since the sterile area does not become hot, the plant material can stay for a longer duration.
3. Bigger flasks having wide lids can be used.

4.1.3.5 Limitations

The airflow velocity can be overcome easily without any strict work practices and aseptic technique; thus, an area of turbulence is created which can introduce room contaminants particles and microorganisms) into the critical work area. A laminar air flow hood Should remain on for 24 hours. If it is turned off; it should be left on for atleast, 30 minutes for its disinfection before use.

4.2 Different Sources of Contamination in an Aseptic Area

There are various contamination sources in an aseptic area, which are discussed below:

1. **Personnel:** Those supervising, performing, or controlling drug manufacturing are a potential source of microbial contamination, due to the following reasons:
   (i) Inadequate training,
   (ii) Direct contact between the hands and starting materials, primary packaging materials, and intermediate or bulk products,
   (iii) Improper hygiene,
   (iv) Unauthorised personnel entering the production, storage, and product control areas,
   (v) Insufficient gowning and protective equipment, and
   (vi) Eating, drinking, or smoking within the storage and processing areas.
2. **Buildings and Facilities:** These are also important contributors to microbial contaminationdue to the following reasons:
   (i) Inadequate size and organisation of the space, which lead to selection errors (such as mix- ups or cross-contamination between consumables, raw materials, in-process materials, and finished products),

(ii) Poor filth and pest controls,

(iii) Rough floors, walls, and ceilings,

(iv) Absence of air filtration systems,

(v) Inadequate lighting and ventilation systems,

(vi) Poorly located vents, ledges, and drains, and

(vii) Improper washing, cleaning, toilet, locker facilities, sanitary operation, and personal cleanliness.

3. **Equipment and Utensils:** These are used during processing, holding, transferring and packaging. They are the common sources of microbial contamination due to the following reasons

(i) Unsuitable design, size, corrosion-causing materials, static material accumulation, and/or adulteration with lubricants, coolants, dirt, and sanitising agents,

(ii) Inadequate cleaning and sanitisation,

(iii) Inefficient cleaning and maintenance due to their designing

(iv) Inappropriate calibration and irregular service, and

(v) Using defective equipment.

4. **Raw Materials:** These are used during production and are considered a potential source ofcontamination due to the following reasons:

(i) Improper storage and handling, which leads to mix-ups or selection errors,

(ii) Microbial or chemical contamination,

(iii) Degradation due to extreme environmental conditions (like heat, cold, sunlight, moisture, etc.),

(iv) Wrong labelling.

(v) Incorrect sampling and testing, and

(vi) Using materials not meeting the acceptance criteria.

5. **Manufacturing Process:** During the manufacturing process, microbial contamination of rawmaterials, intermediates or packaging materials can widely occur due to the following reasons:

(i) Absence of facilities required for manufacturing of a single product,

(ii) Improper cleaning between batches for minimising the amount of product changeovers,

(iii) Use of an open manufacturing system for exposing the product to the room environment,

(iv) Improper zoning,

(v) Lacking an area line clearance (as per the approved procedures) after each cleaning processand between each batch, and

(vi) Lack of cleaning status labelling on all equipment and materials used within the manufacturing facility.

AHVAC (Heating, Ventilation, and Air Conditioning) System: An inappropriate HVACsystem is a possible source of microbial growth and also disperses the contaminants throughout the manufacturing unit. This occurs due to the followlng reasons:

(i) Organic materials accumulate in or near HVAC air intakes,

(ii) Inadequate air filtration system,

(iii) Inadequate magnitude of pressure differentials, which causes flow of reversal,

(iv) Incorrect ratio of fresh air to re-circulated air,

(v) Incapability of accessing ventilation dampers and filtering from outside the manufacturing areas, and

(vi) Non-directional airflow within production or primary packing areas.

4.2.1 Methods of Prevention of Contamination

The steps by which microbial contamination of products can be prevented in aseptic areas arediscussed below:

1. **Personnel:** They can take the following measures:

   (i) Access to production areas by the unauthorised personnel should be restricted, and onlytrained ones should be allowed to enter.

   (ii) Adequate personnel hygiene should be maintained.

   (iii) The personnel should be given proper and regular training with respect to hygiene as well to ensure that their activities do not hamper the product quality.

   (iv) Personnel entering the manufacturing area should wear protective clothing (over-garments, hair cover, beard or moustache cover, and overshoes).

   (v) Personnel should avoid touching with naked hands the exposed products or any part ofequipment in contact with the product.

2. **Facility Design:** This includes the following measures:

   (i) In aseptic rooms, the differential air pressures should be higher than the adjacent controlledareas.

   (ii) Air filtration and air change rates should be set to attain the defined clean room class.

(iii) Unidirectional (laminar flow) air flow should be maintained over critical areas at sufficient velocity to sweep particles away from filling/closing area.

(iv) Ambient temperature and humidity should not be very high.

(v) The ventilated cabinets, RABS (Restricted Access Barrier System), isolators systems, etc. should be used dcpending on the facility/product risk assessment results in order to achieve anabsolute or partial barrier to contain microorganisms at their point of use

(vi) The areas of unequal risk are separated by UV air locks and door barriers.

(vii) All open-container processing should be performed within the isolator/RABS.

(viii) The air pressure of the changing room should be negative with respect to the manufacturing area corridor, but positive with respect to the external adjacent areas.

(ix) The ventilation dampers, specially designed filters, and other services should be positionedsuch that they can be accessed from outside the manufacturing areas (service voids or service corridors) for maintenance purposes.

(x) An impermeable barrier should be used in appropriate areas to prevent cross- contamination between two zones, such as closed systems, pumped, or vacuum transfer of materials.

(xi) HVAC air distribution components should be used for preventing the spreading of contaminants generated within the room.

(xii) All rooms and surfaces should be maintained and monitored for viable and non-viable particulates and this facility should be re-certified on a semi-annual basis.

Facility and equipment design cannot eliminate microbial contamination completely but good risk assessment and consequent hygienic design can reduce these risks several times. For example,

(i) Flow of man and material should be uniform,

(ii) Equipment having smooth surfaces of appropriate material can facilitate effective cleaning,and

(iii) Closed Material Transfer Systems.

3. **Access to Areas:** This includes the following measures:

(i) Access to production, packaging, and QC areas by unauthorised personnel should berestricted.

(ii) Personnel should gain access to these areas only via changıng rooms.

(iii) Materials should be accessed via specific routes (generally air locks).

4. **Building Requirements:** This includes the following measures:
   (i) Smooth, crack-free, and easily cleanable floors, walls, and ceilings should be used as they facilitate easy and effective cleaning.
   (ii) Windows or viewing panels should be closed (non-opening), fixed with wall panels, and sealed to prevent accumulation of dust and microbial contaminants.
   (iii) The designing of pipe work, ventilation, and light points should be such that Creation of recesses which are not easily cleanable is avoided.
   (iv) Sinks of stainless steel should be present within the production areas.
5. **Cleaning and Disinfection:** This includes the following measures:
   (i) Time-to-time cleanliness and disinfection of the areas should be done.
   (ii) Adequate hygiene should be maintained in every aspect of the drug product manufacturing.
   (iii) Cleaning agents of proper grades should be used for minimising health risks.
   (iv) Contact time, application, temperature, mechanical action, and the chemistry of cleaning agents should be considered during the cleaning process.
   (v) The cleaning agents should not be directly applied on the product.
   (vi) The cleaning practices should be validated to prove that the process effectively controlsmicrobial contamination.
6. **Utilities:** This includes the following measures:
   (i) Water of pharmaceutical grade, microbiologically controlled and monitored should be usedin the manufacturing of products.
   (ii) Clean and additive-free steam should be used for cleaning and sanitisation of production tools and equipment, and to supply for autoclaves and humidification.

4.3 CLEAN AREA CLASSIFICATION

The clean or buffer room is the secondary engineering control. It houses the primary engineering controls (the LAFH, BSC, or CA) where the aseptic compounding is actually performed. Clean room is a specially constructed enclosed area, which contains one or more clean zones, where the concentration of airborne particles is controlled using HEPA filters, continuous air circulation, and a physical barrier to non-filtered (or outside) air. Clean rooms establish appropriate environmental levels for airborne particulates, temperature, humidity, air pressure, and airflow patterns. Clean rooms are categorised by their constant air quality or class. Clean rooms are rated as given in table 4.1:

Table 4.1 Classes of Clean Rooms and their Properties.

Clean Room	Properties
Class 10,000 (ISO class 7)	10,000 or less particles of 0.5μ and larger size exist in a given cubic foot of air.
Class 1,000 (ISO class 6)	1,000 or less particles of 0.5 μ and larger size exist in a given cubic foot of air.
Class 100 (ISO class 5)	100 or less particles of 0.5 μ and larger size exist in a given cubic foot of air.

Lower the classification number, cleaner is the air.

Apart from the above-mentioned basic components, a clean room also includes:

1. UV irradiation,
2. Air-lock entry portals,
3. Special filtration or treatment systems for incoming air,
4. Sticky mats for removing particulate matter from shoes, and
5. Positive room air pressure for controlling entry of contaminants from adjacent rooms.

Clean rooms are divided into different classes in standards. Table 4.2 lists the equivalence of classes from different international standards. For manufacturing sterile products, a certain classification (table 4.3) with grades A to D are characterised to activity category (tables 4.3 and 4.4) is used.

Table 4.2 Class Limits for Federal 209D and ISO Standards.

Class		Measured Particle Size (Microeter)					
Federal 209 D	ISO	0.1	0.2	0.3	0.5 (a)	1.0	5.01
1	3	1000	237	102	(1)	8	
10	4	10000	2370	1020	(10)	83	
100	5	100000	23370	10200	(100)	832	29
1000	6	1000000	237000	102000	(1000)	8320	293
10000	7				(10000)	832000	2930
100000	8				(10000)	8320000	293000

(a) - Particle count for this particular size is per ft while others are per m.

Table 4.3 Air Particle Classification System for the Manufacturing of Sterile Products.

GRADE	Maximum Permitted Number of Particles per m Equal to or Above			
	At Rest (b)		In Operation (b)	
	0.5μm (d)	5μm	0.5μm (d)	5μm
A	3500	0	3500	0
B(a)	3500	0	350000	2000
C(b)	350000	2000	3500000	20000
D(c)	3500000	20000	Not defined (c)	Not defined (d)

Remarks

1. In order to reach the air grades B, C, and D, the number of air changes should be related to the room size, and the equipment and personnel in the room. The air system should be providedwith HEPA filters for grades A, B, and C.
2. After 15-20 minutes of "'clean up" period, an unmanned state (no manual activity) should be received.
3. Appropriate alert and action limits should be fixed for particulate and microbiological monitoring results. A corrective action in the operating procedures should be taken in case these limits are exceeded.

The need for other parameters (like temperature, relative humidity, etc.) depends on the nature of product and manufacturing procedure. These parameters do not have any relation with the purifying classes.

Table 4.4 Terminally Sterilised Products.

Grade	Examples of Operation
A	Filling of products, when unusually at risk.
C	Preparation of solutions, when unusually at risk. Filling of product.
D	Preparation of solutions and components for subsequent filling.

Most products should be prepared in grade D environment; while grade C environment shouldbe used in case of an unusual risk.

Table 4.5 Aseptic Parameters.

Grade	Examples of Operation
A	Aseptic preparation and filling
C	Preparation of solutions to be filtered.
D	Handling of components after washing.

The components after washing should be handled in grade D environment. The sterile starting material should be handled in grade A environment with grade B background. Solutions to besterile filtered should be prepared in grade C environment; while if not filtered, the preparation should be done in grade A environment with grade B background. The aseptically prepared products should be handled and filled in grade A environment with grade B background. The sterile ointments, creams, suspensions, and emulsions should be prepared and filled in grade A environment with grade B background, when the product is exposed and is not subsequently filtered. Control of purity of zones by the particles in operation state and microbial control at an aseptic production area is required; and the recommended levels are listed in table 4.6:

Table 4.6 Recommended Limits for Microbial Contamination in the Operation State (Average Values).

GRADE	Air Sample, cfu/m^3	Settle Plates (Diameter 90mm), cfu/4 hours (a)	Contact Plates (Diameter 55mm), cfu/plate	Glove Print, 5 Finger cfu/gloe
A	1	<1	<1	<1
B	10	5	5	5
C	100	50	25	-
D	200	100	50	-

(a) Individual settle plates are exposed for 4 hours or less; cfu - colony-forming unit.

Warning limitation and action for contamination by particles and microbes depend on the controlling results. Also, corrective action should be provided in case of exceeding the above limits.

4.4. MICROBIOLOGICAL ASSAY

4.4.1 Introduction

The microbiological or microbial assay is a type of biological assay in which the relative potency of activity of a compound is determined by measuring the amount required for producing the predicted effect on a suitable test organism under standard conditions.

The principle involved in microbial assays are similar to those applied to assays or higher plants or animals. An existing difference is the relative size of experimental population. In bioassays, the response each test animal produces is observed and results are obtained when afew animals have gone through statistical analysis to calculate mean activity, standard error, etc. In microbial assays, each evaluation is performed using a microbial culture, and the resultsobtained indicate the average response produced by large number of test organisms. Often in bioassays, the log dose and the response have a linear relationship; while in microbial assays; the dose and the response (within certain limits) have a linear relationship.

The microbiological assay is a biological assay performed using microorganisms, e-g. bacteria, yeast, and moulds. These assays are much easier than those performed using mammals for isolating essential vitamin; for example, a growth factor for Lactobacillus proved to be similar to a haematopoietic factor in pernicious anaemic patients.

Many therapeutic agents, such as antibiotics inhibiting microbial growth or the essential growth factors (vitamins and amino acids), are standardised by microbiological assays. The activity of antibiotics (extent of inhibiting the microbial growth), vitamins, or amino acids (extent of supporting the microbial growth) is determined by microbiological assays; while the potency (concentration or amount) of such substances is determined by chemical assays. Thus, microbiological assays of antibiotics, vitamins, and amino acids are significantly important.

4.4.2 Principles

A microbiological assay relies on the principle that when certain compounds are present in limited amounts, the amount of microbial growth corresponds to the amount of these compounds. The basic procedure of most of the microbial assays is same; however, the test conditions vary. The test substance is added to a liquid or gel medium, test microorganism is inoculated on the medium, and the resultant response (which depends on the substance's biochemical effect on the test organism) is observed. It may be a growth response (positive inthe assay of nutrients and negative in the assay of antibiotics), which is determined by counting,optical density, weight, or area; the growth response may be a definite end-point, or an all-or-none response.

In case of either a positive or negative metabolic response, the metabolic products or Changesin some function may be measured. Examples of some measurable metabolic responses are acid production, CO_2 production, oxygen uptake, nitrate reduction, haemolysis of RBCs, anti- luminescent activity, or inhibition of spore germination. In 1962, **Cancellien and Morpurgo** proposed a determination method of amino acids vitamins, and purine and pyrimidine bases. Substances analogous and antagonistic to regular metabolites inhibit the growth of wild, prototrophic strains of bacteria. The nutrilite content can be assayed by adding graded amounts of nutrilite for re-activating the growth.

4.4.3 Merits

***A microbiological assay has the following merits*:**

1. It is suitably used for compounds which cannot be assayed by either physical or chemicalmethods.
2. It is used for the assay of naturally occurring therapeutic agents.
3. It minimises the mortality rate of animals.
4. It is a simple and rapid method as compared to bioassays.
5. It is used for accurate standardisation of medicinal compounds.
6. Tt determines the concentration as well as activity of compounds.
7. It does not require large amount of sample and instruments.
8. Its complete procedure can be automated to minimise the duration.

4.4.4 Demerits

***A microbiological assay has the following demerits*:**

1. It requires a specific test organism for the assay of a particular compound.
2. It demands maintenance of sterile conditions within the laboratory.
3. It may give invalid results due to a slight variation in incubation temperature.
4. It is a time-consuming method.
5. It requires well trained and expert individuals.

4.5 STANDARDISATION OF ANTIBIOTICS/MICROBIOLOGICAL ASSAY OF ANTIBIOTICS

The microbiological assay of an antibiotic is based upon a comparison of the inhibition of growth of micro-organisms by measured concentrations of the antibiotics under examination with that produced by known concentrations of a standard preparation of the antibiotic havinga known activity.

Two general methods are usually employed, the cylinder-plate (or cup plate) method and the turbidimetric (or tube assay) method.

The **cylinder-plate method (Method A)** depends upon diffusion of the antibiotic from a vertical cylinder through a solidified agar layer in a Petri dish or plate to an extent such that growth of the added micro-organism is prevented entirely in a zone around the cylinder containing a solution of the antibiotic. The **turbidimetric method (Method B)** depends upon the inhibition of growth of a microbial culture in a uniform solution of the antibiotic in a fluid medium that is favourable to its rapid growth in the absence of the antibiotic

The assay is designed in such a way that the mathematical model on which the potency equation is based can be proved to be valid. If a parallel-line model is chosen, the two log dose response lines of the preparation under examination and the standard preparation should be parallel; they should be rectilinear over the range of doses used in the calculation. These conditions should be verified by validity tests for a given probability. Other mathematical models, such as the slope ratio method, may be used provided that proof of validity is demonstrated.

4.5.1 Media

Prepare the media required for the preparation of test organism inocula from the ingredients listed in Table 4.7. Minor modifications of the individual ingredients may be made, or reconstituted dehydrated media may be used provided the resulting media have equal or better growth-promoting properties and give a similar standard curve response.

Dissolve the ingredients in sufficient water to produce 1000 ml and add sufficient 1 M sodium hydroxide or 1 M hydrochloric acid, as required so that after sterilization the pH is as given inTable 4.7.

Table 4.7 Media: Quantities in g of ingredients per 1000 ml.

Ingredient	Medium									
	A	B	C	D	E	F	G	H	I	J
Peptone	6.0	6.0	5.0	6.0	6.0	6.0	9.4	-	10.0	-
Pancreatic digest of casein	4.0	-	-	4.0	-	-	-	17.0	-	15.0
Yeast extract	3.0	3.0	1.5	3.0	3.0	3.0	4.7	-	-	-
Beef extract	1.5	1.5	1.5	1.5	1.5	1.5	2.4	-	10.0	-
Dextrose	1.0	-	1.0	1.0	-	-	10.0	2.5	-	-
Papaic digest of soyabean	-	-	-	-	-	-	-	3.0	-	5.0
Agar	15.0	15.0	-	15.0	15.0	15.0	23.5	12.0	17.0	15.0
Glycerin	-	-	-	-	-	-	-	-	10.0	-
Polysorbate 80	-	-	-	-	-	-	-	10.0*	-	-
Sodium chloride	-	-	3.5	-	-	-	10.0	5.0	3. 0	5.0

Table contd...

Dipotassiu mHydrogen Phosphate	-	-	3.68	-	-	-	-	2.5	-	-
Potassium dihydrogen Phosphate	-	-	1.32	-	-	-	-	-	-	-
Final pH (after sterilisation)	6.5-6.6	6.5-6.6	6.95-7.05	7.8-8.0	7.8-8.0	5.8-6.0	6.0-6.2	7.1-7.3	6.9-7.1	7.2-7.4

* Quantity in ml, to be added after boiling the media to dissolve the agar.

4.5.2 Standard Preparation and Units of Activity

A Standard Preparation is an authentic sample of the appropriate antibiotic for which the potency has been precisely determined by reference to the appropriate international standard. The Potency of the standard preparation may be expressed in International Units or in µg per mg of the pure antibiotic.

The Standard Preparations for India are certified by the laboratory of the Indian Pharmacopoeia Commission or by any other notified laboratory(ies) and are maintained and distributed by the agency(ies) notified for the purpose. A Standard Preparation may be replaced by a working standard prepared by any laboratory which should be compared at definite intervals under varying conditions with the standard.

4.5.3 Buffer Solutions

Prepare by dissolving the following quantities given in Table 4.8 of dipotassium hydrogen phosphate and potassium dihydrogen phosphate in sufficient water to produce 1000 ml after sterilisation, adjusting the pH with 8 M phosphoric acid or 10 M potassium hydroxide.

Table 4.8 Buffer Solutions.

Buffer number	Dipotassium Hydrogen Phosphate K_2HPO_4 (g)	Potassium Dihydrogen Phosphate KH_2PO_4 (g)	pH adjusted after sterilisation to
1	2.0	8.0	6.0 ± 0.1
2	16.73	0.523	8.0 ± 0.1
3	-	13.61	4.5 ± 0.1
4	20.0	80.00	6.0 ± 0.1

Table contd...

5	35.0	-	10.5 ± 0.1*
6	13.6	4.0	7.0 ± 0.2

* After addition of 2 ml of 10M potassium hydroxide

4.5.4 Preparation of the Standard Solution

To prepare a stock solution, dissolve a quantityof the Standard Preparation of a given antibiotic, accurately weighed and previously dried where so indicated in Table 4.9, in the solvent specified in the table, and then dilute to the required concentration as indicated. Store in a refrigerator and use within the period indicated.On the day of assay, prepare from the stock solution five or more test dilutions, the successive solutions increasing stepwise in concentration, usually in the ratio 1:1.25 for Method A or smaller for Method B. Use the final diluent specified and a sequence such that the middle or median has the concentration specified in Table 4.9.

Preparation of the Sample Solution: From the information available for the substance under examination (the "unknown"), assign to it an assumed potency per unit weight or volume, and on this assumption prepare on the day of the assay a stock solution and test dilutionas specified for each antibiotic in Table 4.9 but with the same final diluent as used for the Standard Preparation. The assay with 5 levels of the Standard requires only one level of the unknown at a concentration assumed equal to the median level of the standard.4.5.5.

4.5.5 Test Organisms

The test organism for each antibiotic is listed in Table 4.10, together with its identification number in the American Type Culture Collection (ATCC). Maintain a culture on slants of the medium and under the incubation conditions specified in Table 4.11, and transfer weekly to fresh slants.

4.5.6 Preparation of inoculum

Prepare the microbial suspensions for the inoculum for the assay as given in Table 4.11. If the suspensions are prepared by these methods, growth characteristics are sufficiently uniform so that the inoculum can be adequately determined by the trials given below.

Table 4.9 Stock solutions and test dilutions of Standard Preparation.

Antibiotic	Standard Stock Solution					Test Dilution		
	Assay Method	Prior Drying	Initial solvent (further diluent, if different)	Final Stock Concentration per ml	Use before (number of days)	Final diluent	Median dose µg or units per ml	Incubation temp (°C)

Table contd...

Amikacin		No	Water	1 mg	14	Water	10 µg	32-35
Amphotericin B		Yes	DMF[7]	1 mg	Same day	B5	1.0 µg	29-31
Bacitracin		Yes	0.0IM HCl	100 units	Same day	B1	1.0 unit	32-35
Bleomycin		Yes	B6[8]	2 units	14	B6	0.04 units	32-35
Carbenicillin		No	BI	1 mg	14	B6	20 µg	36-37.5
Chlortetracycline		No	0.IM HCl	1 mg	4	Water	2-5 µg	37-39
		No	0.IM HCl	1 mg	4	Water	0.24µg	35-37
Erythromycin		Yes	Methanol	1 mg	14	B2	1-0 µg	35-37
	B A A A		(I0 mg/ml)[9]					
	A A1		(B2)					
	B10A							
Framycetin		Yes	B2	1 mg	14	B2	1.0 µg	30-35
Gentamicin	A A A1 B2AA	Yes	B2	1 mg	30	B2	0.1 µg	36-37.5
Kanamycin sulphate		No	B2	800 units	30	B2	0.8 µnits	37-39
	A A3 B2	No	Water	1000 units	30	Water	10 units	32-35
Neomycin	A A4 A4 B5 A3 B6 B	Yes	B2	1 mg	14	B2	1.0 µg	36-37.5
Novobiocin	B10	Yes	Ethanol	1 mg	5	B4	0.5 µg	32-35
			(10 mg/ml)9					
			(B2)					
Nystatin		Yes	DMF7	1000 units	Same day	B4	20 units	29-31
Oxytetracycline		No	0.IM HCl	1 mg	4	B3	2.5 µg	32-35
		No	0.IM HCl	1 mg	4	Water	0.24 µg	35-37
Polymyxin B		Yes	Water (B4)	10,000 units	14	B4	10 µnits	35-39
Spiramycin		No	Methanol	1mg	1	B2	12-50 units	30-32
Streptomycin		Yes	Water	1mg	30	Water	1-0 µg	32-35
		Yes	Water	1mg	30	Water	30 µg	35-37

Table contd...

Tetracycline		No	0.IM HCl	1mg	1	Water	2-5 µg	32-35
		No	0.IM HCl	1mg	4	Water	0.24 µg	35-37
Tobramycin		Yes	Water	1mg	14	Water	2-5 µg	32-35
Tylosin		No	*	1mg	Same day	*	0.05 - 0.25	37
							units	

With Bacillus pumilus ATCC 14884 as test organism; 2. With Staphylococcus aureus ATCC 29737 as test organism;3. With Bacillus cereus var mycoides ATCC 11778 as test organism;4. With Bacillus subtilis ATCC 6633 as test organism; 5. With Klebsiella pneumoniae ATCC 10031 as test organism;6. With Staphylococcus aureus ATCC 29737 as test organism; 7. DMF = Dimethyl formamide 8. In columns 4 & 7, B denotes buffer solution and the number following refers to the buffer number in Table 4.8; 9. Initial concentration of stock solution, 10. With Staphylococcus aureus ATCC 9144 as test organism.

NOTES: For Amphotericin B and Nystatin, prepare the standard solutions and the sample test solutionsimultaneously.

For Amphotericin B, further dilute the stock solution with dimethyl formamide to give concentrations of 12.8,16,20,25, & 31.2µg per ml prior to making the test solutions. The test dilution of the sample prepared from the solution of the substance under examination should contain the same amount of dimethyl formamide as the test dilutions of the Standard preparation.

For Bacitracin, each of the standard test dilutions should contain the same amount of hydrochloric acid as the testdilution of the sample.

For Nystatin, further dilute the stock solution with dimethyl formamide to give concentrations of 64.0, 80.0, 100.0,125.0,156.0 µg per ml prior to making the test dilutions. Prepare the standard response line solutions simultaneously with dilution of the sample being examined. The test dilution of the sample prepared from the solution of the substance being examined should contain the same amount of dimethyl formamide as test dilutionsof the Standard Preparation. Protect the solutions from light.

When making the stock solution of Polymyxin B, add 2 ml of water for each 5 mg of the weighted Standard preparation material.

Where indicated, dry about 100 mg of the Standard Preparation before use in an oven at a pressure not exceeding 0.7 kPa at 60° for 3 hours, except in the case of Bleomycin (dry at 25° for 4 hours), Novobiocin (dry at 100° for 4hours), Gentamicin (dry at 110° for 3hours) and Nystatin (dry at 40° for 2 hours),

Where two level factorial assays are performed use the following test doses per ml: Amphotericin B, 1.0 to 4.0 µg; Bacitracin, 1.0 to 4.0 units; Kanamycin Sulphate, 5.0 to 20.0 units; Streptomycin, 5.0 o 20.0 µg

Table 4.10 Test Organisms for Microbiological Assay of Antibiotics.

Antibiotic	Test Organism	ATCC[1] No.
Amikacin	*Staphylococcus aureus*	29737
Amphotericin B	*Saccharomyces cerevisiae*	9763
Bacitracin	*Micrococcus luteus*	10240
Bleomycin	*Mycobacterium smegmatis*	607
Carbenicillin	*Pseudomonas aeruginosa*	25619
Chlortetracycline	*Bacillus pumilus*	14884
Erythromycin	*Micrococcus luteus*	9341
Framycetin	*Bacillus pumilus*	14884
	Bacillus subtilis	6633
Gentamicin	*Staphylococcus epidermidis*	12228
Kanamycin sulphate	*Bacillus pumilus*	14884
Antibiotic	**Test Organism**	**ATCC[1] No.**
	Staphylococcus aureus	29737
Neomycin	*Staphylococcus epidermidis*	12228
Novobiocin	*Staphylococcus epidermidis*	12228
Nystatin	*Saccharomyces cerevisiae*	2601
Oxytetracycline	*Bacillus cereus var mycoides*	11778
	Staphylococcus aureus	29737
Polymyxin B	*Bordetella bronchiseptica*	4617
Spiramycin	*Bacillus pumilus*	6633
Streptomycin	*Bacillus subtilis*	6633
	Klebsiella pnumoniae	10031
Tetracycline	*Bacillus cereus*	11778
	Staphylococcus aureus	29737
Tobramycin	*Staphylococcus aureus*	29737
Tylosin	*Staphylococcus aureus*	9144

1. American Type Culture Collection, 21301 Park Lawn Drive, Rockville, MD20852, USA

4.5.7 Determination of Inoculum

For Method A. After the suspension is prepared as given under Table 4.11, add different volumes of it to each of several different flasks containing 100 ml of the medium specified in Table 4.9 (the volume of suspension suggested in Table 4.9 may be used as a guide). Using these inocula, prepare inoculated plates as described for the specific antibiotic assay. While conducting cylinder-plate assays, double-layer plates may be prepared by pouring a seed layer (inoculated with the desired micro-organism) over a solidified uninoculated base layer. For each Petri dish, 21 ml of base layer and 4 ml of the seed layer may be generally suitable. Fill each cylinder with the median concentration of the antibiotic (Table 4.9) and then incubate the plates. After incubation, examine and measure the zones of inhibition. The volume of suspension that produces the optimum zones of inhibition with respect to both clarity and diameter determines the inoculum to be used for the assay.

For Method B. Proceed as described for Method A and, using the several inocula, carry out the procedure as described for the specific antibiotic assay running only the high and low concentrations of the standard response curve. After incubation, read the absorbances of the appropriate tubes. Determine which inoculum produces the best response between the low and high antibiotic concentrations and use this inoculum for the assay.

Table 4.11 Preparation of inoculum.

Test organism	Incubation conditions			Suggested dilution factor	Suggested inoculum composition		
	Medium/ Method of Preparation	Tem (°C°)	Time		Medium	Amount (ml per 100 ml)	Antibiotics assayed
Bacillus cereus var. mycoides	A 1/2	32-35	5 days	-	F	As required	Oxytetracycline Tetracycline
Bacillus pumilus	A 1/2	32-35	5 days	-	D	As required	Chlortetracycline Framycetin Kanamycin sulphate
Bacillus subtilis	A 1/2	32-35	5 days	-	EEB A	As required As required As required As required	Framycetin Kanamycin B Spiramycin Streptomycin
Bordetella bronchiseptica	A/1	32-35	24 hr	1:20	H	0.1	Polymyxin B
Klebsiella pneumoniae	A/1	36-37	24 hr	1:25	C	0.1	Streptomycin

Table contd...

Micrococcus luteus (9341)	A/1	32-35	24 hr	1:40	D	1.5	Erythromycin
Micrococcus luteus (10240)	A/1	32-35	24 hr	1:35	A	0.3	Bacitracin
Mycobacterium smegmatis	J/4	36-37.5	48 hr	As determined	I	1.0	Bleomycin
Pseudomonas aeruginosa[2]	A/1	36-37.5	24 hr	1:25	H	0.5	Carbenicillin
Saccharomyces cerevisiae (9763)	G/3	29-31	48 hr	As determined	G	1.0	Amphotericin B
Saccharomyces cerevisiae (2601)	G/3	29-31	48 hr	As determined	G	1.0	Nystatin
Staphylococcus aureus (29737)	A/1	32-35	24 hr	1:20	C	0.1	Amikacin Doxycycline Oxytetracycline Tetracycline Tobramycin Tylosin
					C	0.2	Kanamycin sulphate
Staphylococcus epidermidis	A/1	32-35	24 hr	1:40		0.03	Gentamicin
					D DA	0.4	Neomycin
						4.0	Novobiocin

1. Use Medium A containing 300 mg of manganese sulphate per litre.
2. For Pseudomonas aeruginosa in the assay of Carbenicillin, use the dilution yielding 25 per cent light transmission, rather than the stock suspension, for preparing the inoculum suspension.

Methods of preparation of test organism suspension:

1. Maintain the test organism on slants of Medium A and transfer to a fresh slant once a week. Incubate the slants at the temperature indicated above for 24 hours. Using 3 ml of saline solution, wash the organism from the agar slant onto a large agar surface of Medium A such as a Roux bottle containing 250 ml of agar. Incubate for 24 hours at the appropriate temperature. Wash the growth from the nutrient surface using 50 ml of

saline solution. Store the test organism under refrigeration. Determine the dilution factor which will give 25 per cent light transmission at about 530 nm. Determine the amount of suspensions to be added to each 100 ml of agar of nutrient broth by use of test plates or test broth. Store the suspension under refrigeration.

2. Proceed as described in Method 1 but incubate the Roux bottle for 5 days. Centrifuge and decant the supernatantliquid. Resuspend the sediment with 50 to 70 ml of saline solution and heat the suspension for 30 minutes at 70°. Wash the spore suspension three times with 50 to 70 ml of saline solution. Resuspend in 50 to 70 ml of saline solution and heat- shock again for 30 minutes. Use test plates to determine the amount of the suspension required for 100 ml of agar. Store the suspension under refrigeration.
3. Maintain the test organism on 10 ml agar slants of Medium G. Incubate at 32° to 35° for 24 hours. Inoculate 100 ml of nutrient broth. Incubate for 16 to 18 hours at 37° and proceed as described in Method I.
4. Proceed as described in Method 1 but wash the growth from the nutrient surface using 50 ml of Medium 1 (prepared without agar) in place of saline solution.

4.5.8 Apparatus

All equipment is to be thoroughly cleaned before and after each use. Glassware for holding andtransferring test organisms is sterilised by dry heat or by steam.

Temperature Control. Thermostatic control is required at several stages of a microbial assay,when culturing a microorganism and preparing its inoculum and during incubation in a plate assay. Closer control of the temperature is imperative during incubation in a tube assay whichmay be achieved by either circulated air or water, the greater heat capacity of water lending it some advantage over circulating air.

Spectrophotometer: Measuring transmittance within a fairly narrow frequency band requires a suitable spectrophotometer in which the wavelength of the light source can be varied or restricted by the use of a 580-nm filter for preparing inocula of the required density or with a 530-nm filter for reading a absorbance in a tube assay. For the latter purpose, the instrument may be arranged to accept the tube in which incubation takes place, to accept a modified cell fitted with a drain that facilitates rapid change of contents, or preferably fixed with a flow- through cell for a continuous flow-through analysis. Set the instrument at zero absorbance with clear, uninoculated broth prepared as specified for the particular antibiotic, including the same amount of test solution and formaldehyde as found in each sample.

Cylinder-plate assay receptacles: Use rectangular glass trays or glass or plastic Petri dishes (approximately 20 x 100 mm) having covers of suitable material and assay cylinders made of glass, porcelain, aluminium or stainless steel with outside diameter 8 mm ± 0.1 mm, inside diameter 6mm ± 0.1mm and length 10 mm ± 0.1 mm. Instead of cylinders, holes 5 to 8 mm in diameter may be bored in the medium with a sterile borer, or paper discs of suitable quality paper may be used. Carefully clean the cylinder to remove all residues. An occasional acid bath, e.g. with about 2 M nitric acid or with chromic acid solution is needed.

Turbidimetric assay receptacles: For assay tubes, use glass or plastic test-tubes, e.g. 16 mm x 125 mm or 18 mm x 150 mm that are relatively uniform in length, diameter, and thickness and substantially free from surface blemishes and scratches. Cleanse thoroughly to remove allantibiotic residues and traces of cleaning solution and sterilise tubes that have been used previously before subsequent use.

4.5.9 Assay Designs

Microbial assays gain markedly in precision by the segregation of relatively large sources of potential error and bias through suitable experimental designs. In a cylinder plate assay, the essential comparisons are restricted to relationships between zone diameter measurements within plates, exclusive of the variation between plates in their preparation and subsequent handling. To conduct a turbidimetric assay so that the difference in observed turbidity will reflect the differences in the antibiotic concentration requires both greater uniformity in the environment created for the tubes through closer thermostatic control of the incubator and theavoidance of systematic bias by a random placement of replicate tubes in separate tube racks, each rack containing one complete set of treatments. The essential comparisons are then restricted to relationships between the observed turbidities within racks. Within these restrictions, two alternative designs are recommended; i.e. a 3-level (or 2-level) factorial assay, or a 1- level assay with a standard curve. For a factorial assay, prepare solutions of 3 or 2 corresponding test dilutions for both the standard and the unknowns on the day of the assay, asdescribed under Preparation of the Standard and Preparation of the samples. For a 1-level assay with a standard curve, prepare instead solutions of five test dilutions of the standard and a solution of a single median test level of the unknown as described in the same sections. Consider an assay as preliminary if its computed potency with either design is less than 60 percent or more than 150 per cent of that assumed in preparing the stock solution of the unknown.In such a case, adjust its assumed potency accordingly and repeat the assay.

Microbial determinations of potency are subject to inter-assay variables as well as intra-assay variables, so that two or more independent assays are required for a reliable estimate of the potency of a given assay preparation or unknown. Starting with separately prepared stock solutions and test dilutions of both the standard and unknown, repeat the assay of a given unknown on a different day. If the estimated potency of the second assay differs significantly, as indicated by the calculated standard error, from that of the first, conduct one or more additional assays. The combined result of a series of smaller, independent assays spread over a number of days is a more reliable estimate of potency than that from a single large assay withthe same total number of plates or tubes.

4.5.10 Methods

Carry out the microbiological assay by Method A or Method B.

A. Cylinder-plate or Cup-plate method

Inoculate a previously liquefied medium appropriate to the assay (Tables 1 and 3) with the requisite quantity of suspension of the micro-organism, add the suspension to the medium at a temperature between 40° and 50° and immediately pour the inoculated medium into the petri dishes or large rectangular plates to give a depth of 3 to 4 mm (1 to 2mm for nystatin). Ensure that the layers of medium are uniform in thickness, by placing the dishes or plates on a level surface.

Store the prepared dishes or plates in a manner so as to ensure that no significant growth or death of the test organism occurs before the dishes or plates are used and that the surface of theagar layer is dry at the time of use.

Using the appropriate buffer solutions indicated in Tables 4.8 and 4.9, prepare solutions of known concentrations of the standard preparation and solutions of the corresponding assumedof concentrations the antibiotic to be examined. Where directions have been given in the individual monograph for preparing the solutions, these should be followed and further dilutions made with buffer solution as indicated in Table 4.9. Apply the solutions to the surfaceof the solid medium in sterile cylinders or in cavities prepared in the agar. The volume of solution added to each cylinder or cavity must be uniform and sufficient almost to fill the holes when these are used. When paper discs are used these should be sterilised by exposure of both sides under a sterilising lamp and then impregnated with the standard solutions or the test solutions and placed on the surface of the medium. When Petri dishes are used, arrange the solutions of the Standard Preparation and the antibiotic under examination on each dish so that, they alternate around the dish and so that the highest concentrations of standard and test preparations are not adjacent. When plates are used, place the solutions in a Latin square design, if the plate is a square, or if it is not, in a randomised block design. The same random design should not be used repeatedly.

Leave the dishes or plates standing for 1 to 4 hours at room temperature or at 4°, as appropriate,as a period of preincubation diffusion to minimise the effects of variation in time between theapplication of the different solutions. Incubate them for about 18 hours at the temperature indicated in Table 4.9. Accurately measure the diameters or areas of the circular inhibition zones and calculate the results. Selection of the assay design should be based on the requirements stated in the individual monograph. Some of the usual assay designs are as follows.

(a) One-level assay with standard curve

Standard Solution: Dissolve an accurately weighed quantity of the Standard Preparation of the antibiotic, previously dried where necessary, in the solvent specified in Table 4.9, and then dilute to the required concentration, as indicated, to give the stock solution. Store in a refrigerator and use within the period indicated. On the day of the assay prepare from the stocksolution, 5 dilutions (solutions S1 to S5) representing 5 test levels of the standard and increasing stepwise in the ratio of 4:5. Use the diluent specified in Table 4.9 and a sequence such that the middle or median has the concentration given in the table.

Sample Solution: From the information available for the antibiotic preparation which is being examined (the "unknown") assign to it an assumed potency per unit weight or volume and on this assumption prepare on the day of the assay a stock solution with same solvent as used forthe standard. Prepare from this stock solution a dilution to a concentration equal to the medianlevel of the standard to give the sample solution.

Method: For preparing the standard curve, use a total of 12 Petri dishes or plates to accommodate 72 cylinders or cavities. A set of 3 plates (18 cylinders or cavities) is used for each dilution. On each of the three plates of a set fill alternate cylinders or cavities with solutionS3 (representing the median concentration of the standard solution) and each of the remaining9 cylinders or cavities with one of the other 4 dilutions of the standard solution. Repeat the process for the other 3 dilutions of the standard solution. For each unknown preparation use a set of 3 plates (18 cylinders or cavities) and fill alternate cylinders or cavities with the sample solution and each of the remaining 9 cylinders of cavities with solution S3. Incubate the plates for about 18 hours at the specified temperature and measure the diameters or the zones of inhibition.

Estimation of potency: Average the readings of solution S3 and the readings of the concentration tested on each set of three plates, and average also all 36 readings of solution S3. The average of the 36 readings of solution S3 is the correction point for the curve. Correctthe average value obtained for each concentration (S1, S2, S4 and S5) to the figure it would be if the readings for solution S3 for that set of three plates were the same as the correction point. Thus, in correcting the value obtained with any concentration, say S1, if the average of 36 readings of S3 is, for example, 18.0 mm and the average of the S3 concentrations on one set ofthree plates is 17.8 mm, the correction is + 0.2 mm. If the average reading of S1 is 16.0 mm the corrected reading of S1 is 16.2 mm. Plot these corrected values including the average of the 36 readings for solutions S3 on two-cycle semilog paper, using the concentrations in

Units or µg per ml (as the ordinate logarithmic scale) and the diameter of the zones of inhibitionas the abscissa. Draw the straight response line either through these points by inspection or through the points plotted for highest and lowest zone diameters obtained by means of the following expressions:

where,

$$L = \frac{3a + 2b + c - e}{5}; \quad H = \frac{3e + 2d + c - a}{5}$$

L = the calculated zone diameter for the lowest concentration of the standard curve response line.

H = the calculated zone diameter for the highest concentration of the standard curve response line.

c = average zone diameter of 36 readings of the reference point standard solution.

a, b, d, e = corrected average values for the other standard solutions, lowest to highest concentrations, respectively.

Average the zone diameters for the sample solution and for solutions S3 on the plates used forthe sample solution. If sample gives a large average zone size than the average of the standard(solution S3), add the difference between them to the zone size of solution S3 of the standard response line. If the average sample zone size is smaller than the standard values, subtract the difference between them from the zone size of solution S3 of the standard response line. Fromthe response line read the concentration corresponding to these corrected values of zone sizes.From the dilution factors the potency of the sample may be calculated.

(b) **Two-level factorial assay:** Prepare parallel dilutions containing 2 levels of both the standard (S1 and S2) and the unknown(U1and U2). On each of four or more plates, fill each of its four cylinders or cavities with a different test dilution, alternating standard and unknown. Keep the plates at room temperatureand measure the diameters of the zones of inhibition.

Estimation of potency. Sum the diameters of the zones of each dilution and calculate the percentage potency of the sample (in terms of the standard) from the following equation:

Per cent potency = Antilog (2. 0 + a log I)

wherein 'a' may have a positive or negative value and should be used algebraically and

$$a = \frac{(U_1 + U_2) - (S_1 + S_2)}{(U_1 - U_2) + (S_1 - S_2)}$$

U1 and U2 are the sums of the zone diameters with solutions of the unknown of high and lowlevels.

S1 and S2 are the sums of the zone diameters with solutions of the standard of high and lowlevels.

I = ratio of dilutions.

If the potency of the sample is lower than 60 per cent or greater that 150 per cent of the standard,the assay is invalid and should be repeated using higher or lower dilutions of the same solution.

The potency of the sample may be calculated from the expression 100

$$\textbf{Potency of the sample} = \frac{\textbf{per cent potency x assumed Potency of the sample}}{\textbf{100}}$$

(c) Other designs

100

1. Factorial assay containing parallel dilution of three test levels of standard and the unknown.
2. Factorial assay using two test levels of standard and two test levels of two differentunknowns.

B. Turbidimetric or Tube assay method

The method has the advantage of a shorter incubation period for the growth of the test organism(usually 3 to 4 hours) but the presence of solvent residues or other inhibitory substances affects this assay more than the cylinder plates assay and care should be taken to ensure freedom fromsuch substances in the final test solutions. This method is not recommended for cloudy or turbid preparations.

Prepare five different concentrations of the standard solution for preparing the standard curve by diluting the stock solution of the Standard Preparation of the antibiotic (Table 4.9) and increasing stepwise in the ration 4:5. Select the median concentration (Table 4.9) and dilute thesolution of the substance being examined (unknown) to obtain approximately this concentration. Place 1 ml of each concentration of the standard solution and of the sample solution in each of the tubes in duplicate. To each tube add 9 ml of nutrient medium (Table 4.9) previously seeded with the appropriate test organism (Table 4.9).

At the same time prepare three control tubes, one containing the inoculated culture medium (culture control), another identical with it but treated immediately with 0.5 ml of dilute formaldehyde solution (blank) and a third containing uninoculated culture medium.

Place all the tubes, randomly distributed or in a randomized block arrangement, in an incubatoror water-bath and maintain them at the specified temperature (Table 4.9) for 3 to 4 hours. Afterincubation add 0.5 ml of dilute formaldehyde solution to each tube. Measure the growth of thetest organism by determining the absorbance at about 530 nm of each of the solutions in the tubes against the blank.

Estimation of potency: Plot the average absorbances for each concentration of the standard on semi-logarithmic paper with the absorbances on the arithmetic scale and concentrations on the logarithmic scale. Construct the best straight response line through the points either by inspection or by means of the following expressions:

$$L = \frac{3a + 2b + c - e}{5}; \quad H = \frac{3e + 2d + c - a}{5}$$

where,

L = the calculated absorbance for the lowest concentration of the standard response line.

H = the calculated absorbance for the highest concentration of the standard response line.

a, b, c, d, e = average absorbance values for each concentration of the standard response linelowest to highest respectively.

Plot the values obtained for L and H and connect the points. Average the absorbances for the sample and read the antibiotic concentration from the standard response line. Multiply the concentration by the appropriate dilution factors to obtain the antibiotic content of the sample.

4.5.11 Precision of Microbiological Assays

The fiducial limits of error of the estimated potency should be not less than 95 per cent and notmore than 105 per cent of the estimated potency unless otherwise stated in the individual monograph.

This degree of precision is the minimum acceptable for determining that the final product complies with the official requirements and may be inadequate for those deciding, for example, the potency which should be stated on the label or used as the basis for calculating the quantity of an antibiotic to be incorporated in a preparation. In such circumstances, assays of greater precision may be desirable with, for instance, fiducial limits of error of the order of 98 per centto 102 per cent. With this degree of precision, the lower fiducial limit lies close to the estimatedpotency. By using this limit, instead of the estimated potency, to assign a potency to the antibiotic either for labelling or for calculating the quantity to be included in a preparation, there is less likelihood of the final preparation subsequently failing to comply with the officialrequirements for potency.

4.5.12 Methods for Standardisation of Vitamins

Vitamins are essentially required for the growth and multiplication of microorganisms (whichare highly sensitive even to small amounts of growth factors). These test microorganisms can synthesis the factor being assayed which forms the basis of microbiological assay of vitaminsand amino acids. The test microorganisms used for the standardisation of water-soluble vitamins are given in table 4.12.

Table 4.12 Test Microorganisms and Conditions for the Microbial Assay of Vitamins.

Vitamins	Test Microorganisms	Incubation Temperature (⁰C)	Assay pH
Vitamin B12	*Lactobacillus leichamannii ATCC 7830*	37	6.1
	Poteriochromonas stipitata ATCC 11532	30	5.5
Vitamin B6	*Saccharomyces uvarum ATCC 9080*	30	4.5
	Tetrahymena thermophila ATCC 30008	30	6.1
Vitamins	**Test Microorganisms**	**Incubation Temperature (⁰C)**	**Assay pH**
Riboflavin	*Lactobacillus casei ATCC 7469*	37	6.8
	Tetrahymena thermophila ATCC 30008	30	6.1
Thiamine	*Lactobacillus viridescens ATCC 12706*	30	6.0
	Ochromonas danica ATCC 30004	30	5.5
Biotin	*Lactobacillus plantarum ATCC 8014*	37	6.8
	Ochromonas danica ATCC 30004	30	5.5
Niacin	*Lactobacillus plantarum ATCC 8014*	37	6.8
	Tetrahymena thermophila ATCC 30008	30	6.1
Pantothenate	*Lactobacillus plantarum ATCC 8014*	37	6.7
	Tetrahymena thermophila ATCC30008	30	6.1

4.5.12.1 Principle

Vitamins are essential growth factor for microorganisms. In the standardisation of vitamins, the ability of test organisms to use the substance being standardised under a proper nutritional condition is measured. These growth factors (vitamins) are required by the organisms in micro or nano grams. The growth response produced by the test organism is proportional to the amount of growth factor added to the medium.

4.5.12.2 Standardisation of Calcium Pantothenate

The reagents and the methods utilised for the standardisation of calcium pantothenate are discussed below:

Reagents

Standard Stock Solution of Calcium Pantothenate

The stock solution is prepared by dissolving 50mg calcium pantothenate in 500ml water. To the resultant solution, 10ml of 0.2N acetic acid and 100ml of 1.6%w/v sodium acetate solution are added. Volume is adjusted up to 1000ml by adding water. This solution is stored in a refrigerator under toluene. Each ml of this resultant stock solution contains 50ug of calcium pantothenate.

Standard Solution

Each ml of standard solution contains 0.04ug of calcium pantothenate. This solution is preparedby diluting the standard stock solution with water.

Test Solution

The concentration of calcium pantothenate in test solution is approximately equivalent to thatin the standard solution prepared in water.

Medium

The medium utilised contains the following ingredients:

Ingredients	Amounts
Acid-hydrolysed casein solution	25 ml
Cystine- tryptophan solution	25 ml
polysorbate 80 solution	0.25 ml
Dextrose (anhydrous)	10gm
Sodium acetate (anhydrous)	5gm
Adenine-guanine-uracil solution	5ml
Riboflavin-thiamine HCl-biotin solution	5ml
P-amino benzoic acid-niacin-pyridoxine HCl solution	5ml
Salt solution A	5ml
Salt solution B	5ml

The medium is prepared by dissolving the anhydrous dextrose and sodium acetate in previously mixed solutions. The pH of solution is adjusted to 6.8 using 1 N NaOH. Ultimately, the solutionis diluted to 250ml with water and mixed.

Stock Culture of Organism

The stock culture is prepared by dissolving 2gm water-soluble yeast extract in 100ml water; 500mg each of anhydrous dextrose and sodium acetate, and 1.5gm agar is also added. The resultant mixture is heated to dissolve the agar. 10ml of this hot solution is added to test tubesand sterilised at 121°C by mounting in vertical position. Stab culture of Lactobacillus plantarum is prepared in 3 tubes, incubated for 16-24 hours at 30-37 ^{0}C and stored in a refrigerator.

Preparation of Inoculum

The inoculum is prepared by transferring cells from the stock culture of organism to 10ml of culture medium in a sterile tube, and then incubating for 16-24 hours at 30-37°C.

Principle

Pantothenate assay medium (a dehydrated medium) is free from pantothenic acid or pantothenate, but contains other essential nutrients and vitamins used for preparing the cultureof L. plantarum. Addition of calcium pantothenate in increasing concentrations as specified yields a growth response which is either turbidimetrically or titrimetrically measured.

Procedure

1. Standard solution in 1, 2, 3, 4, and 5ml is added to test tubes in duplicate.
2. Each of these tubes and another four similar tubes containing no standard solution are addedwith 5ml medium solution and volume is adjusted to 10ml with water.
3. Volumes of test solution corresponding to 3 or more of the levels as taken above are addedto similar test tubes, in duplicate.
4. Each tube is added with 5ml medium solution and volume is adjusted up to 10ml with water.
5. A complete set of standard and assay tubes is placed in a tube rack and the duplicate set is kept in the other rack.
6. Tubes of both the series are autoclaved for 5 minutes at 121°C. After cooling, a drop of inoculum is added to each tube except 2 of the 4 tubes which do not have standard solution (un-inoculated blanks), mixed, and incubated for 16-24 hours at 30-37° C.
7. Spectrophotometer is used to measure the transmittance of the tubes at a specific wavelengthlying between 540-660nm.

Calculation

A standard concentration-response curve 1s obtained by plotting the transmittance against the logarithm of the ml of standard solution per tube. The response is calculated by summing the two transmittances for each level of the test solution. This curve helps in determining the concentration of calcium pantothenate in the test sample.

4.5.12.3 Standardisation of Niacin

The selected organism should have the ability to utilise free niacin, niacinamide, nicotinuric acid, cozymase, and niacinamide nucleoside. This requirement is satisfied by Lactobacillus plantarum (an acid forming organism), cannot synthesise niacin for its metabolic processes. This bacterium is also non-pathogenic, can be easily cultured, and is negligibly affected by stimulatory or inhibitory substances present in niacin-containing pharmaceutical preparations.

This organism is grown on a simple stab culture containing gelatin, yeast extract, and glucose.For assay it is cultured in assay tubes by transferring to the liquid medium containing the basicmedium having an optimum amount of added niacin. A measurable response can range from 0.05-0.5μg of niacin per tube.

For preparing the niacin test solution, sample is extracted, either in acid or alkali medium by adding such amount of alkali or acid that each ml of final volume contains 0.1gm niacin.

Reagents

1. **Standard Niacin Stock Solution I:** It contains 100ug/ml of U.S.P. Niacin RS.
2. **Standard Niacin Stock Solution II:** It contains 10ug/ml of U.S.P. Niacin RS, and isprepared by diluting solution I with water.
3. **Standard Niacin Solution**: It contains 10-40ng of niacin per ml and is prepared by dilutingsolution with water.
4. **Basal Medium Stock Solution:** It contains the following ingredients:

Ingredients	Amounts
Acid-hydrolysed casein solution Cystine-tryptophan solution Dextrose (anhydrous) Sodium acetate (anhydrous) Adenine-guanine-uracil solution Riboflavin-thiamine hydrochloride-biotin solution Aminobenzoic acid-calcium pantothenate-pyridoxineHydrochloride solution Salt Solution ASalt Solution B	25 ml25 ml 10gm 5 gm 5 ml 5 ml 5 ml5 ml5 ml

The medium is prepared by dissolving anhydrous dextrose and sodium acetate in the previouslymixed solutions. The pH is adjusted to 6.8 using 1N NaOH solution, and volume is adjusted to250ml by adding water.

Culture Medium

The culture medium is prepared in a series of test tubes each containing 5ml of basal medium stock solution. Further, each tube is added with 5ml water containing 1.0ug of niacin, pluggedwith cotton, autoclaved at 121°C for 15 minutes, and cooled

Preparation of Inoculum

The inoculum is prepared by transferring cells from the stock culture of Lactobacillus plantarum to 10ml culture medium in a sterile tube, and then incubating for 16-24 hours at 30-37°C.

Principle

Niacin assay medium (a dehydrated medium) is free from nicotinic acid and its analogues, but contains other essential nutrients and vitamins used for preparing the culture of L. plantarum. Addition of nicotinic acid or its analogues in increasing concentrations as specified yields a growth response which is either turbidimetrically or titrimetrically measured.

Procedure

1. The spectrophotometer is calibrated as per the Pharmacopoeia.
2. Standard niacin solution in 0.0, 0.5, 1.0, 1.5, 2.0, 5.0 ml is added to test tubes in duplicate.
3. Each tube is added with 5ml of basal medium stock solution and volume is adjusted to 10mlwith water.
4. Each tube is added with 5ml medium solution and volume is adjusted up to 10ml with water.
5. Tubes containing the material to be assayed are prepared by taking in duplicate, 1.0, 2.0,3.0, and 4.0 ml, respectively of the test solution of the material to be assayed.
6. Again each tube is added with 5ml basal medium stock solution and volume is adjusted upto 10ml with water.
7. The contents in tubes are mixed, plugged with cotton, and autoclaved.
8. After cooling, each tube is aseptically inoculated with a drop of inoculum and incubated for16-24 hours at 30-37°C.
9. The transmittance for the un-inoculated blank is adjusted at 1.0, using which the transmittance of inoculated blank is read.
10. Finally, using the transmittance of the inoculated blank set at 1.0, the transmittance for theremaining tubes is measured.

Calculation

A standard curve of niacin standard transmittances for each level of standard niacin solution isplotted against μg of niacin present in the respective tubes. By interpolating this standard curve,the niacin content of test solution in each tube is determined. The niacin content of the test material is calculated from the average values obtained from at least 6 tubes not varying by more than tl0% from the average. For expressing the results as niacinamide, the obtained valuesare multiplied by 0.992.

4.5.12.4 Standardisation of Vitamin B12 Assay Preparation

1. An accurately weighed quantity of the material to be assayed is taken in the form of finepowder in a vessel.
2. An aqueous extracting solution is prepared containing 1.29gm disodium phosphate 1.1gm anhydrous citric acid, and 1.0gm sodium meta bisulphite in each 100ml,
3. For each gm or ml of material taken, 25ml of this freshly prepared aqueous extractingsolution is added and mixed.
4. The resultant mixture is autoclaved at 121°C for 10 minutes.
5. The undissolved particles of the extract are allowed to settle, and later filtered or centrifuged.
6. An aliquot of this so obtained clear solution is diluted with water so that the final test solutioncontains vitamin B12 having activity equivalent to the standard cyanocobalamin solution addedto the assay tubes.

Basal Medium Stock Solutions

The basal medium utilised contains the following ingredients given in table 4.13:

Table 4.13 Basal Medium Ingredients.

Ingredients	Amounts
L-Cystine	0.1 gm
L-Tryptophan	0.05 gm
1N Hydrochloric acid	5 ml
Adenine-guanine-uracil solution	5 ml
Xanthine solution	5 ml
Vitamin solution I	10 ml
Vitamin solution II	10 ml
Salt solution A	5 ml
Salt solution B	5 ml
Asparagine solution	5 ml
Acid-hydrolysed casein solution	25 ml
Dextrose (anhydrous)	10 gm

Table contd...

Sodium Acetate (anhydrous)	5 gm
Ascorbic Acid	1 gm
Polysorbate 80 Solution	5 ml

Cysteine and tryptophan are dissolved in hydrochloric acid and then the next 8 solutions are added. To the resultant solution, 100ml water is added and mixed. To this mixture, dextrose, sodium acetate, and ascorbic acid are added. The solution is filtered and polysorbate 80 solutionis added. The pH is adjusted between 5.5 and 6.0 using 1 N sodium hydroxide, and volume is adjusted to 250ml with purified water.

Standard Cyanocobalamin Stock Solution

The standard stock solution is prepared by adding sufficient amount of 25% alcohol to an accurately weighed quantity of U.S.P. cyanocobalamin RS. The solution obtained having a known concentration of 1.0 μgm of cyanocobalamin per ml is stored in a refrigerator.

Standard Cyanocobalamin Solution

A fresh standard cyanocobalamin solution is prepared for each assay. It is prepared by diluting a suitable volume of standard cyanocobalamin stock solution with water up to a measured volume such that after incubation the difference in transmittance between the inoculated blank and 5.0ml of the standard cyanocobalamin solution is not less than that which corresponds to a difference of 1.25mg in a dried cell weight. This concentration falls between 0.01-0.04μg/mlof standard cyanocobalamin solution.

Culture Medium

The culture medium is prepared by dissolving 0.75gm water-soluble yeast extract, 0.75gm dried peptone, 1.0gm of anhydrous dextrose, and 0.20gm of potassium biphosphate in 60-70ml of water. To the resultant solution, 10ml tomato juice and 1ml polysorbate 80 solution are added. The pH of the solution is adjusted to 6.8 using 1N NaOH solution, and volume is adjusted to 100ml with water. 10ml portions of the solution are taken in test tubes, plugged with cotton, and autoclaved at 121°C for 15 minutes. The solution is immediately cooled to avoid colour formation which may result due to overheating of the medium.

Suspension Medium

The suspension medium is prepared by diluting a measured volume of basal medium stock solution using an equal volume of water. 10ml portions of this diluted medium are taken in testtubes, sterilised, and cooled same as for the culture medium.

Stock Culture of Lactobacillus Leichmannii

1. The stock culture of the organism is prepared by heating with continuous stirring of 100ml of culture media with 1.0-1.5gm of agar medium on a steam bath till the agar dissolves.
2. Approximately, 10 ml portions of the hot solution are taken in test tubes, plugged with cotton,and autoclaved at 121°C for 15 minutes.
3. After cooling the tubes in a vertical position, 3 or more tubes are inoculated by transferring stab of a pure culture of Lactobacillus Leichmannii.
4. The inoculum is incubated for 16-24 hours at 30-40 ± 0.5°C temperature, and stored in a refrigerator.
5. Fresh stab cultures are prepared at least thrice a week, and are not used for inoculum preparation if more than four days old.
6. The microorganism activity can be increased by transferring daily or twice-daily the stab culture to the point where definite turbidity in the liquid inoculum can be observed after 2-4 hours of inoculation.
7. A Slow-growing culture rarely yields a suitable response curve, resulting in irregular results.

Preparation of Inoculum

1. The inoculum is prepared by transferring cells from the stock culture of organism to two steriletubes, each containing 10ml culture medium.
2. These culture tubes are then incubated for 16-24 hours at 30-40 ± 0.5°C temperature.
3. The incubated tubes are aseptically centrifuged, and the supernatant is decanted.
4. The cells from the culture are suspended and mixed with 5ml sterile suspension medium.
5. The volume is adjusted using sterile suspension medium so that 1 in 20 dilutions in saline TS produces 70% transmittance on a spectrophotometer at 530nm wavelength, and read againstsaline TS set at 100% transmittance.
6. 1 in 400 dilution of the adjusted suspension is prepared using basal medium stock solution to use for the test inoculum.

Principle

Vitamin B12 assay medium is free from vitamin B12, but contains other essential nutrients and vitamins used for the culture of *Lactobacillus leichmannii*. Addition of U.S.P. cyanocobalamin reference in increasing concentrations as specified yields a standard curve providing growth response which is either titrimetrically or turbidimetrically measured.

Procedure

1. Standard cyanocobalamin solution in 1.0ml, 1.5ml, 2.0ml, 3.0 ml, 4.0ml, and 5.0ml is added to thoroughly cleaned hard-glass test tubes in duplicate.
2. These tubes and other 4 1dentical empty tubes are added with 5.0 ml of basal medium stocksolution and volume is adjusted to 10ml with water.
3. Assay preparation in 1.0ml, 1.5ml, 2.0ml, 3.0ml, and 4.0ml is added to similar tubes in duplicate.
4. Each of these tubes is added with 5ml basal medium solution and volume is adjusted to 10mlwith water.
5. A complete set of standard and assay tubes is placed in a tube rack and the duplicate set is placed in the other rack in random order.
6. The tubes are covered to prevent bacterial contamination and autoclaved for 5 minutes at 121°C.
7. The tubes are immediately cooled to prevent colour formation which may result due to overheating of the medium.
8. Each tube [except 2 of the 4 without standard cyanocobalamin solution (the un- inoculated blanks)] are added with 0.5ml inoculum.
9. These tubes are incubated for 16-24 hours at 30-40±0.5°C temperature. Bacterial growth isterminated by heating for 5 minutes at temperature not lower than 80°C.
10. After cooling to room temperature, the contents are agitated, and when a steady state 1s reached, transmittance is recorded in a spectrophotometer at the wavelength of 30nm. This steady state is observed after a few seconds of agitation when the reading remains unchanged for 30 seconds or more.
11. Reading for each tube is recorded after the same time interval.
12. With the transmittance set at 100% for the un-inoculated blank, the transmittance of the inoculated blank is recorded. If the difference is greater than 5% or if Contamination with a foreign microorganism is observed, the assay results are ignored.
13. With the transmittance set at 100% for the un-inoculated blank, the transmittance of the remaining tubes is recorded. If the slope of the standard curve indicates a sensitivity problem, the assay results are ignored.

Calculation

1. For preparing a standard concentration-response curve, any abnormal individual transmittance is prevented.
2. For each level of the standard, the response is calculated by adding the duplicate values of the transmittances ($\sum$) as the difference, $y = 2.00 - \sum$.

3. On plotting this response against the logarithm of the ml of standard cyanocobalamin solution per tube, a straight line or a smooth curve is produced.
4. The response (y) is calculated by adding the two transmittances for each level of the assay preparation.
5. From the standard curve the logarithm of the volume of standard preparation correspondingto each value of y falling within the range of the lowest and highest points plotted for the standard is determined.
6. From this logarithm value the logarithm of the volume (ml) of assay preparation is subtracted to obtain the difference (x) for each dosage level.
7. Average the values of x for each of three or more dosage levels to obtain x = M (the log- relative potency of assay preparation).
8. The quantity of U.S.P. Cyanocobalamin RS (μg) corresponding to the cyanocobalamin in the material being standardised is determined by the equation:

   Antilog M = antilog (M + log R)

Where, R Number of μg of cyanocobalamin present in each mg of the material standardised.

4.5.13 Standardisation of Amino Acids

Microbiological assays were used for quantitation of amino acids since many years as they were the most reliable, sensitive, and specific available tests. They can be used for any type ofbiological material, however sometimes they are affected by the activators or inhibitors present in the material being standardised. These inexpensive methods are used for analysing large batches of samples, but are time-consuming and also not suitable for all amino acids.

Amino acids are essential for the growth and replication of some microorganisms. Many strainsof such microbes depend on a particular amino acid. Thus, if such microorganisms are culturedusing a small amount of that particular amino acid, a limited degree of growth will be observed, which is measured by turbidimetry or by measuring the increased lactic acid production by either microtitration or pH change.

Guthrie and Susi introduced a modified version of microbiological assay utilising diffusion in gels in clinical biochemistry laboratories for screening blood Samples having increased phenylalanine levels. This test was named as the Guthrie test (after its inventors) and is the most widely used microbiological assay method of an amino acid. This bacterial inhibition assay is based on the ability of phenylalanine to counteract the effects of β-2-

theienylalanine (a competitive metabolic antagonist on the growth of a special strain of Bacillussubtilis which de pends on phenylalanine for its growth

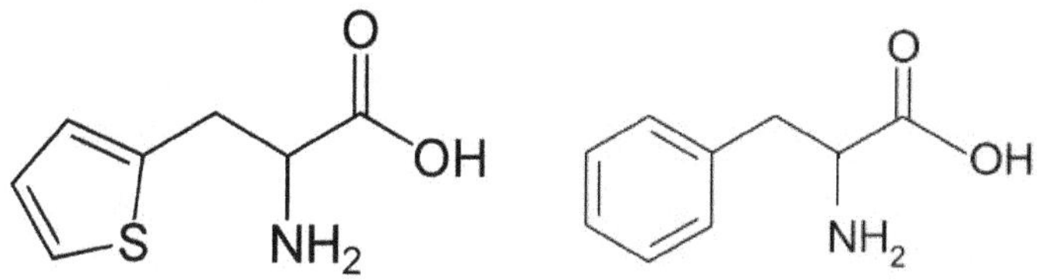

Fig.4.5 β-2-Thienylalanine Phenylalanine.

Figure 4.5: Guthrie Test: The similarity in structure between phenylalanine and its metabolic antagonist β-2-thienylalanine provides the basis for a microbiological assay for phenylalanine.

The test is carried out on an agar layer in which a mixture of the suspension of B. subtilis spores, minimum amount of growth nutrients, and a fixed amount of β-2 thienylalanine is added.

Filter paper discs of 4 mm diameter are soaked in blood and placed on the agar surface along with the blood-soaked discs of phenylalanine standards. These agar plates are incubated at 37°C overnight. Bacterial growth is observed only when phenylalanine concentration in the blood discs is sufficient to overcome the effects of β-2 thienylalanine. Growth is observed in zones of growth around each disc. The next day diameter of each zone of growth is measured and related to phenylalanine concentration.

4.6 ASSESSMENT OF A NEW ANTIBIOTIC

Antimicrobial Resistance (AMR) occurs when microbes (bacteria, viruses, fungi, and parasites) change in ways making the medications used for curing the infections ineffective. Ifnew antib1otics are not introduced, the patients will die due to the previously treatable infections.

However, a major issue is adequate evaluation or the antibiotics, particularly by payers and/orHealth Technology Assessment (HTA) Bodies, to take account of AMR and reflect the full benefit provided to patients and society.

Two Key Challenges

1. Clinical trials are designed for establishing non-inferiority, while HTA bodies requiredemonstration of clinical superiority.
2. HTA bodies do not have a mechanism to evaluate the health benefits of antibiotics, andcontrol the rise in AMR.

Elements of Value Relevant to Antibiotics: these are given in the table below 4.14 and explained as follows.

Table 4.14 Additional Elements of Value Relevant to Antibiotics.

Relevant Benefits included in Traditional HTA	Other Types of Benefit of Possible relevance to Antibiotics
Health gain Unmet need Cost offsets Productivity benefits	Insurance value Diversity value Diagnostic value Uniqueness or innovation value Enablement value Spectrum value

Relevant Benefits included in Traditional HTA: are

Health Gain

1. It includes life extension and quality of life gains.
2. It is accepted as a criterion for positive HTA recommendation.
3. Evidence required by HTA bodies is often inaccessible for antibiotics (superiority trials).

Unmet Need

1. It includes severity of disease and current availability of alternative treatments.
2. It involves use of priority pathogen lists.

Cost Offsets

1. It includes the reduction in costs in other areas as a result of use of new medicine.
2. It involves use of modelling studies and/or evidence from clinical trials.

Productivity Benefits

1. It involves profits or losses related to value of patient's time, receiving medical care or out of work.
2. It involves use of modelling studies and/or evidence from clinical trials/observational studies.

Other Types of Benefit of Possible relevance to Antibiotics: are

Insurance Value

1. It is the value of treatment available in case of catastrophic health events, e.g, outbreak of MDR infections which cannot be controlled by existing last-line antibiotics.

2. It is analogous to availability of a fire engine.
3. It also needs to add in the "precautionary principle".
4. It involves use of modelling studies.

Diversity Value

1. It is the selection pressure, i.e., the antibiotic is able to eliminate susceptible species of bacteria but no other resistant pathogens; thus these pathogens survive and multiply, making the antibiotic ineffective.
2. It involves evidence that reducing selection pressure by withdrawing antibiotic for a periodof time may result in restoration of susceptibilities.
3. It involves use of modelling studies.

Diagnostic Value

1. If infection is diagnosed at an early stage, appropriate antibiotic therapy can be started earlier.
2. It needs evidence of test accuracy.

Uniqueness or Innovation Value

1. It is the potential value associated with new or unique mechanism of action.
2. Antibiotics with novel mechanism of action may avoid problems of cross-resistanceoccurring in many existing classes.
3. Discovery of new mechanism of action of an antibiotic makes it easier for' follow on' products to enter market.
4. It needs evidence of new mechanism of action.

Enablement Value

1. It is the availability of effective antibiotics supporting many surgical procedures and treatments for people having compromised immune systems.
2. It involves use of modelling studies.

Spectrum Value

1. Narrow spectrum antibiotics may be more valuable than broad spectrum ones as the formercan reduce spread of AMR by preventing 'collateral damage' to the microbiome.
2. It depends on the antibiotic.

Reasons for which additional elements of value for antibiotics are required:

Given below are the reasons for which additional elements of value for antibiotics are required:

1. **AMR is a Public Health Priority:** The rise of AMR is a serious threat, control of which is a priority for the national and international health organisations. The current HTA methods donot account for the value of reducing this public health threat, e.g., of the insurance value of having a treatment available in case of a future major or rapidly intensifying resistance problem.
2. **Diverse Set of Non-Inferior Antibiotics is Valuable to Society**: Since AMR is increasing widely, it has become valuable developing a new antibiotic for MDR pathogens, even if it is ineffective than the existing antibiotics in treating susceptible (non-resistant) pathogens. This concept is unique to antibiotics and is not considered by HTA bodies.
3. **Non-Clinical and Microbiology Data are important for Demonstrating the Value of Antibiotics:** Non-clinical and microbiology data for antibiotics can predict their results. Due to the difficulties in conducting clinical trials for antibiotics for MDR pathogens, regulators accept these alternative types of evidence as part of the approval process in areas of high unmetneed.
4. **Antibiotics have Benefits that go Beyond the Patient Treated:** When one patient is treatedwith an antibiotic, the spread of the infectious disease is reduced thus benefitting the population.
5. **Antibiotics Enable Other Types of Treatment and Procedures:** Apart from treating infections, antibiotics also reduce the risk associated with other types of treatment such as surgery and chemotherapy.

UNIT V

Microbial Contaminants and Cell Culture

Spoilage:

Spoilage is chemical and physicochemical degradation of pharmaceutical products rendering it unsuitable for use. Spoilage is not desirable in pharmaceutical industry because deterioration of drugs and excipient occurs, as a result product may lose its quality and it may become ineffective. Entire batch may be required to be discarded. This may cost huge lose to the manufacturer. Moreover, it may attract litigation from the consumers which may cause huge financial loss to the Company. Damaged products may damage reputation of the manufacturing company which may attract further financial loss. Microbial spoilage may present potential health hazards to the consumers like toxicity, infection or even death. Toxic metabolites may be produced due to microbial growth which may cause health hazards. Microbes may deteriorate drugs and thereby reduce potency of the medicament. There could be change in the appearance of the product like decolorization, phase separation, and odour formation etc. Following types of microbial spoilage occurs in pharmaceutical products.

1. **Chemical spoilage.**
2. **Physicochemical spoilage**
3. **Biological spoilage.**

Chemical Spoilage - Chemical spoilage means deterioration of chemical nature of drugs and excipients. Molecular structure of the ingredients may change. This change may affect physicochemical properties of the preparation. Potency of the drug may decrease. Further microbial growth may occur if chemical degradation of preservative occurs. Similarly, chemical degradation of surfactants, organic polymers etc, may damage specialized micro-environment for which they are used. Along with microbial contamination some - chemicals may also cause chemical spoilage like pesticide, disinfectants, bleaching agent, sanitizer etc. may add to chemical spoilage.

Physicochemical spoilage - This type of spoilage may change physico-chemical properties of product. Following types of changes may occur.

i. Viable growth - Viable growth of microbes may occur inside the container. The growth may be visible in the form of floating layers, turbidity, hemps, etc. Contamination of products by fungus species like Aspergillus sp. may cause this type spoilage. Some bacterial species may also show viable growth.

ii. Gas production -Some microbes may produce gas inside the containers. These gases may be visible in the form of bubbles, floccules etc. Contamination of products with bacteria like E. coli may produce gas if it contains sugars.

iii. Colouration / Decolouration -Some microbes may decolourise formulation or it may produce unique colour which is different from the normal colour of the product.

iv. Odour formation-Microbial growth in the finished product may produce bad odour or characteristic odour. It may produce a characteristic rotten smell.

v. Taste change -Microbial spoilage may change the taste of the oral formulations. It may impart bitter or obnoxious taste to the oral formulation.

Biological Spoilage - Spoilage of pharmaceuticals may produce some undesirable and dangerous molecule which has undesirable biological effects. Some microbes may produce toxins, pyrogens or other harmful metabolites. These biomolecules may be present in the product from the very beginning. Spoilage may occur, although no microbial contamination was there.

Factors affecting the microbial Spoilage of the Pharmacultad products.

There are so many factors which affects Microbial spoilage. Some of these factors reduce rate of spoilage where as some factors increases the rate of spoilage. These factors are related to nutritional requirement of micro-organisms, environment and nature of micro-organism. These factors must be studied to minimise the impact of spoilage.

Following factors affect the microbial spoilage of Pharmaceutical products.

i) **Number of contaminating micro-organism -** There may not be sufficient spoilage if number of contaminants are less. This low level it contaminants may not able to multiply due to design of the formulation. However during long storage these microbes may cause damage. If initial contamination is high then it may present an undesirable challenge. Products will be damaged quickly due to presence of high numbers of microbes. High level of contamination occurs due to lapses in manufacturing process or due to high loads of contaminants in raw materials.

ii) **Type of micro-organism -** Some microorganisms are more aggressive than others. They can quickly multiply and spoilage is much faster. However, aggressive microbes may not multiply initially due to presence of preservative and other substances. Contamination of product with natural communities of non-aggressive micro-organism can facilitate growth of other aggressive contaminants.

iii) **Presence of nutrients -** In product Micro-organism can utilise formulation components as nutrients and utilise these components for biosynthesis and growth. Many formulations may contain crude animal, vegetable and microbial products which creates a conducive environment for microbial growth and subsequent spoilage. Additives like sugar, amino acid, polyhydric alcohol may act as microbial nutrients. Primary contaminants may produce metabolites which could be used by aggressive microbes as nutrient. Demineralised water which is prepare by ion-exchange resins may contain nutrients.

iv) **Presence of water -** Presence of water in formulation may promote microbial growth and subsequent spoilage. Uncomplexed water or free excess water promotes this spoilage. Presence of free water may be measured by water activity. It is a ratio between 'vapour pressure of formulation and vapour pressure of water in similar condition'. If water activity is 1 then it is conducive for microbial growth. Chances of microbial growth decreases with decrease in value of water activity. A value less than 0.88 is considered safe to prevent spoilage. However, some microbes can grow in extremely low water value condition. - Aspergillus glaucus can grow at a water activity value of 0.61.

v) **Oxidation-reduction potential-** Contaminating micro-organism may requires terminal electron accepter to facilitate functioning respiratory pathway. Presence of dissolved oxygen increases redox potential of the product thereby promote microbial growth and spoilage.

vi) **Temperature -** Storage temperature is a great controller of microbial growth and spoilage. However, spoilage may occur over a range -20oC to 60oC. Microbial growth and spoilage is less in low temperature and high temperature. Storing products at a cool place (8oC to 12oC) may cause negligible spoilage. High temperature can also prevent spoilage. Water for injection is stored above 80oC before filling and sealing. So extreme temperature can minimise spoilage.

vii) **pH-** Microbes prefer neutral pH for their growth. However, some microbes may prefer slightly acidic pH. Extremely acidic or alkaline pH of the formulation may prevent microbial growth and subsequent spoilage. Some communities of microbes can survive in extreme pH and change the pH, thereby support growth of other micro-organism.

viii) **Containers and packaging -** Chances of contamination in single dose ampoules and vials are negligible. However multidose containers be contaminated by users themselves. Change in designs of these containers may minimize contamination and spoilage. Wide mouthed containers for creams and ointments are replaced by narrow mouthed tubes with screw cap closures. Multidose injections are stored in containers which has self-sealing rubber wads. Containers are sealed such a way so that it can prevent entry of water and oxygen to minimise water activity and redox potential.

ix) **Presence of protection materials -** Some materials in formulation may protect microbes during sterilisation process. Polymers like gelatin, starch etc., may increase microbial resistance to heat. Microbes may get adsorbed in particles and become more resistant to heat. Source and types of microbial contaminants. Microbes are very important part of our environment. They are present almost anywhere and everywhere. So, contamination may occur to pharmaceutical products in large scale manufacturing, in small scale hospital manufacturing or during use by the patient.

x) **Following are the different source of microbial contamination in pharmaceutical products. In large scale manufacturing: -** In large scale manufacturing as well as medium and small-scale manufacturing contamination may occur from following sources. Water -Water is a major source of contamination. Common water borne micro-organism like Pseudomonas, Achromo bacteria and other low demand gram negative groups are present in portable water as well as in purified water. Ion-exchange column may be contaminated by water source and micro-organism may multiply there to contaminate purified water. Water which is purified by reverse osmosis process may also be contaminated if osmosis membrane is no properly disinfected. Even distilled water may also be contaminated if it is stored for few days at normal temperature.

Raw materials - Pharmaceutical products are prepared from varieties of raw materials. Clays and earth materials like bentonite, kaolin etc may contain anaerobia spores like Clostridium sp. Starch may contain coliform bacteria like E. Coli. Gums may contain actinomycetes. Animal Products may contain a variety of bacterial like E. coli, Salmonella sp etc. Air of the manufacturing area: Air is filled with billions of suspending particles and microbes. Fungus spores, like penicillium, mucor, aspergillus etc. Bacterial spores like Bacillius sp. etc., are also present. These spores and micro-organism may contaminate pharmaceutical products. This type of contamination is minimised by practice of manufacturing in clean room and in aseptic room under continuous flow of sterile air through HEPA filter. Personnel- manufacturing staff may also contaminate pharmaceutical products. Personnel may be infected with various types of infections like coliform bacteria, staphylococci, streptococci, Actino bacteria, Candida. These types of contamination may be minimised by pooper health check-up, vaccination and hygiene of the personnel. Protective gear and pooper training of the personnel may also minimise the contamination. Equipment - Equipment of manufacturing may contain microbes if it is not sterilized properly. Grinder, blender, filter etc., may contain non-specific and local communities of micro-organism.

Containers: containers may cause contamination if it is not sterile. In hospital manufacturing - In hospital manufacturing water and environment are the major source of contaminants. In hospitals, water is stored in storage tank which may develop fungus, bacteria and algae type of microbes. Hospital air may be contaminated with pathogenic microorganism due to the presences of infected patients and numerous visitors. Herman source Pharmaceutical products may be contaminated during use. Patient may self-contaminate his medicine. Contaminants may travel to other patients through doctors, nurses etc.

Preservation of pharmaceutical products using antimicrobial agents: Antimicrobial agents are those substances which can kill of inhibit growth of micro-organism. These antimicrobial agents are included in formulation in order to minimize levels of contaminated micro-organism.

These antimicrobial agents are called preservatives. These preservatives can generally prevent or kill low levels of contamination. Preservatives are not used in those formulations which has low risk of contamination and subsequent microbial growth. Formulations which contain high level of acid, alkali, sugar etc., may not require preservative. Formulations of antibiotics and other anti-microbial substances may not require preservative.

A good preservative should have following characteristics. It should be a *broad spectrum antimicrobial agent*, i.e. it should be effective against variety of microorganisms. However, most active preservatives are ineffective against some microbes. A good preservative *should have a fast killing and inhibition rate and it should selectively react with contaminants and it should not react with ingredients of the formulation.* However, most preservatives interact with ingredients of the formulations. A good preservative should be *non-irritant and non-toxic* to the patients. However, many preservative have toxic effects and cause irritation of skin when used in formulation for topical application. Some preservatives even cause contact dermatitis. A good preservative should be *stable and it should remain active throughout the shelf-life of the product.* However effectiveness of the preservative may change depending upon so many factors. Concentration of preservatives determine efficacy of its preservation power. Antimicrobial activity of preservative increases with the concentration. Activity of phenol decreases 64 times if concentration is halved. Antimicrobial activity of preservative is also dependent on storage temperature. Decrease in storage temperature may reduce killing activity of preservative. It may be calculated by determining temperature co-efficient. Preservative which is used in formulation may not be available for antimicrobial activity. An unstable equilibria is formed between preservative and available preservative which controls mass of micro-organism.

Unavailable preservative helps to maintain equilibria by constantly supplying available molecule. Availability of preservative may also decrease with increased solute concentration and decrease water activity. Ionic and weakly acidic preservatives exhibit their antimicrobial activity when they are not ionised. They produce maximum activity when ionisation is very low. Preservative may distribute itself depending on its affinity in a multiphase system. It may distribute itself in water phase and oil phase by an unstable equilibrium. Parameters like partition coefficient, polymer binding constant and oil-water ratio must be considered while using a preservative in a formulation. Packaging material can interfere with preservation activity of preservative. Preservative may leach, permeate and interact with rubber, plastic, cork etc. Different types of preservatives are used in pharmaceutical products. Acid, alkali and esters are used as preservative. *Benzoic acid* is used as preservative. Its sodium salt, *sodium benzoate* is also used as preservative. Its ester *methyl hydroxybenzoate* is also used as preservative. Some alcohols like *chlorobutol, benzyl alcohol* etc are used as preservative. Some phenolic compounds like *phenol, chlorocresol* etc are also used as preservatives. Some mercuric compounds, such as *thiomersal* etc are used as preservative. Many other compounds like *benzalkonium chloride, cetrimide* are used as preservative. Even compounds like *chloroform and formaldehyde* can be used as preservative.

Assessment of microbial contamination and Spoilage: Assessment of microbial content of a pharmaceutical product is very essential. Sterile product should be perfectly free from micro-organism and that can be assessed by a test of sterility. However, non-sterile products may contain some micro-organisms. These micro-organisms could be pathogenic and non-pathogenic. All these micro-organisms can cause spoilage and may cause potential health hazards. Number of total micro-organisms present in a product must be low and should be within permissible limit.

Types and nature of the microbes should also be assessed to determine the presence of specific microbes. *Total number of microbes and types of microbes is assessed by microbial limit test.* Following tests are performed to assess the microbial contamination and subsequent spoilage. **1. Test of sterility**-. Indian pharmacopoeia, British pharmacopoeia and United States pharmacopoeia recommends test of sterility for some pharmaceutical products. Procedure is similar with little variations. Indian pharmacopoeia recommended tests are discussed briefly. Two methods are there i.e., direct inoculation and membrane filtration.

i) Direct inoculation- In this method, little amount of sample is directly added to the culture media which was specified in pharmacopeia. This inoculated media is then incubated for specified period of time. Presence of growth indicates the presence of microorganism which is sourced from sample. Hence it may be concluded that sample is not sterile. Sample may be termed sterile in absence of any growth.

ii) Membrane filtration- In this method sample is filtered through a membrane filter and washed with diluting fluid. Microbes, if present, will be there at the top of the filter paper. Now this filter paper is inoculated into specified culture media. If growth is observed then it indicates that product is not sterile. A positive and negative control test must also be conducted in both the above-mentioned method.

Microbial limit test:

The European pharmacopoeia recommends both qualitative and quantitative assessment of micro-organism.

United States Pharmacopoeia recommends microbiological Limit test. It has two parts,

(i) Total Aerobic microbial count and

(ii) Test for specified microorganism.

(i) Total Aerobic microbial count

In this method specified amount of test sample (10gm) is taken and mixed with specified amount (90ml) of peptone water. This is sample dilution. There are specific procedure to make dilutions for water insoluble products and fatty products. Total microbial count is examined by following procedure- First, examination of sample by membrane filtration method- 10 ml of prepared dilution is mixed with 90 ml of peptone water and filtered through membrane filter. It is then washed 3 times with sterile peptone water. One filter paper is placed in petridish containing Soyabean Caesin Digest Agar media and incubated for 5 days at 30-35oC. Bacterial count is determined by counting colonies. Another filter paper is placed in Sabouraud Dextrose Agar Media and incubated for 5 days at 20-25oC. Fungal count is then determined.

Second, Examination of sample **plate count method**- In this method prepared dilution is directly transferred to 4 petridishes. Two for bacteria and two for fungus. In first two petridishes 15 ml of Soyabean Caesin Digest Agar media is added. Colonies are counter after incubation for 5 days at 30-35oC. In remaining two petridishes 15 ml of Sabouraud Dextrose Agar Media was transferred and incubated at 20-25oC. Colonies are counted.

(ii) Test for specified micro-organism

Specific identification tests for Escherichia coli, Salmonella, Pseudomonas aeruginea and Staphylococcus aureus is performed. *E. coli is cultivated in Mac Conkes agar* media. Colonies are identified by characteristics metallic shine. *Salmonella are cultivated on bismuth sulphite agar media* and identified by black or green colonies. *Pseudomonas aeruginosa is identified by cultivating in cetrimide agar media.* Colonies slow greenish colour. *Staphylococcus aureus is caltivated in Vogel Johnson agar media* and identified by black colonies surround by yellow zones.

Periodic test- Periodic test of the product for total microbial count must be done in order to determine continuing efficacy of the product. Many alternative tests may be done for detection and determination of micro-organism e.g., Luciferase test, Epifluorescence, electrical impedance etc.

Evaluation of microbial stability of formulation.

Microbial stability of a formulation is dependent on effectiveness of its preservative. Chemical assay and biological assay may assure effectiveness of preservative but it may lose its activity due to presence of other ingredients in the formulation. Some formulations do not require preservative because they act as self-preservative. Some formulation does not require preservative because it contains antimicrobial agents like antibiotics as ingredient. Some formulation may contain high sugar concentration, salt concentration and may act as **self-preservative.** So, the ability of the formulation to protect itself from microbial growth must ascertain to determine microbial stability of the formulation. It is done by preservative efficacy test.

Basic principle of this test is to *inoculate products with different types of specified microorganism with specific quantity. Little amount of inoculated product is removed at a specific interval. Then viable count of this withdrawn sample is determined.* United States Pharmacopoeia, European Pharmacopoeia etc recommends this type of tests. *The concentration of the test organism should be 105 -106 cells per ml or gm. Total microbial count is performed in 0 hr, 6 hrs, 24 hrs, 48 hrs. 7 days, 14 days and 28 days.* British pharmacopeia recommends test even after 28 days. Different bacterial species are used for this purpose. They are *Staphylococcus aureus, Pseudomonus aeruginosa and E. coli.* Different fungus species are also used. They are *Candida albicans, Aspergillus niger* etc.

Animal cell culture

Animal cell culture is a microbiological technique in which animal cells and tissues are obtained and maintained in a suitable environment. It is further divided into,

Organotypic: Animal Organ Tissue Culture & **Histotypic**: Animal Cell Culture.

Animal cells can be grown only up to certain generations. Their growth requires typical conditions and a physicochemical environment. Animal cell culture prepared from collecting tissue or cells from an organism is called a "**Primary culture**." The sequence of subcultures prepared from primary culture is called "**Cell lines**".

Animal cell cultures can be divided into two distinct groups depending on the number of cell divisions occurring during the process;

1. Primary cell culture

Primary cell culture is the first culture obtained directly from animal tissue via mechanical and chemical disintegration or enzymatic methods. The cells of the primary cell culture are slow-growing cells that carry all characteristics of the original tissue or cells. Since these cultures are obtained directly from the origin, they have the same number of chromosomes as the original cells.

Primary cell cultures are performed in order to preserve and maintain the growth of cells on an artificial growth medium at a particular condition.

Primary cell cultures can be sub cultured to obtained other cultures that either continue to grow indefinitely or die after a few subcultures. The subsequent subculture of primary cell culture results in the introduction of mutations into the cells, which might result in cell lines.

The morphology of cells in the primary cell cultures might be different and varied, with the most commonly observed morphological structures being epithelium type, epithelioid type, fibroblast type, and connective tissue type. Primary cell cultures are difficult to obtain and usually have a shorter lifespan. Besides, these are prone to contamination by bacteria and viruses. The increase in cell numbers in the primary cell culture can result in exhaustion of the substrate and nutrients, which affects cellular activity. Usually, primary cell cultures need to be subcultured in order to maintain continuous cell growth once they reach the confluence stage.

Primary cell cultures can be further divided into two groups depending on the kind of cells present in the culture;

a. Anchorage-dependent/Adherent cells

The cells in the culture require a stable biologically inert surface for adherence and growth. The surface should be solid and nontoxic as these cells are difficult to grow as cell suspensions. These cells are usually obtained from the tissues of organs where the cells remain immobilized within the connective tissue. Examples of adherent cells include kidney cells and mouse fibroblast STO cells.

b. Anchorage-independent/ Suspension cells

These cells can grow efficiently as cell suspensions and do not require a solid surface for attachment. These can be grown on liquid media continuously to obtain fresh subcultures.

The ability of the cells to grow as suspension depends on the source of cells as cells that remain as suspensions in the body are effective suspension cells.

Examples of suspension cells include blood cells that are vascular and remain suspended in the plasma.

2. Secondary cell culture

Secondary cell cultures are obtained after the primary cell cultures are subsequently sub cultured over a period of time in fresh culture media. The cells of the secondary cell cultures are long-lasting as these have a higher lifespan due to the availability of appropriate nutrients at regular intervals of time. Secondary cell cultures are favored over primary cell cultures as these are more readily available and are easy to grow and preserve. These are formed from the enzymatic treatment of the adherent cells followed by washing and resuspension of cells in particular volumes of fresh media.

Secondary cell cultures are prepared when the number of cells in the primary culture exceeds the capacity of the medium to support growth. Secondary cultures help to maintain an optimal cell density necessary for continued growth. The cells of the secondary cell culture might not resemble that on the parental tissue as mutations, and genetic alterations might be introduced during the subculture process. The cells can be transformed as, in some cases, the continuous subculture can lead to immortal cells.

The risk of contamination by bacteria and viruses is less as the cells transform and become less susceptible to infections. An important disadvantage associated with secondary cell culture is that the cells might develop the tendency to differentiate over a long period of time and result in aberrant cells.

Cell Lines

A cell line is a group of cells that are formed from the subculture of primary culture consisting of a pure culture of cells. Cell lines usually display functional features that are close to the primary cells, but the genotype and phenotype of the cells can be modified. A cell line consists of several cell lineages with similar or different phenotypes. Cell lines can be further divided into two groups based on the growth patterns of the cells;

Finite cell lines

Finite cell lines are cell lines where the cells in the culture divide for a limited number of times, after which they eventually die. The cells in the finite cell lines can divide from 20 to 100 times before they eventually die and cannot divide anymore. The number of cell division and lifespan depends on a number of factors like cell lineage differences, species, culture conditions, and media. The cells of the finite cell lines grow as adherent cells on solid surfaces.

Continuous cell lines

Continuous cell lines are cells that exhibit indefinite growth via subsequent subcultures. The cells in the continuous cell lines grow faster to form an independent culture. The cells are immortal and can divide indefinitely. The cells in the continuous cell lines can be transformed via genetic alterations and are also tumorigenic.

The transformed cells are formed from the normal primary cell cultures after treatment with chemical carcinogens or by infection with oncogenic viruses. The cells are capable of growing to prepare higher cell density and can grow as suspensions on liquid media. These cells can even grow on top of each other to form multilayered structures on the culture vessels.

Examples of common Cell Lines

The following are some of the common examples of cell lines;

a. HeLa cell line

- HeLa cells are one of the first continuous culture human cell lines with the help of cells of the cervical carcinoma.
- These cells are used for processes like virus cultivation and preclinical drug evaluation.

b. HL 60 (Leukemia)

c. MCF-7 (breast cancer cells)

Procedure or Protocol of Animal cell culture

1. Growth Conditions

Animal cell culture requires the use of specific culture media that are more complex and specific than the basic culture media used for microbial growth. Some of the important basic components of the media are inorganic salts, nitrogen source, energy source, vitamins, fat and fat-soluble vitamins, growth factors, and hormones. In some cases, pH buffering systems and antibiotics are also added. The temperature for the growth depends on the source of the cell as different organisms require different temperatures for cell growth and division. Warm-blooded animal cells can be cultured at 37°C as the optimal temperature, whereas cold-blooded animals grow between 15°C-25°C.

2. Primary cell culture

Primary cell cultures are obtained from fresh tissues that are removed from the organs with the help of an aseptic razor. In some cases, the cells are removed by the use of chemical disintegrators or proteolytic enzymes. The cell suspension obtained is washed with buffering liquid in order to remove the proteolytic enzymes. The cell suspension is poured onto a flat surface which can be a culture vessel or a sterile Petri plate. The cells that can adhere to the base of the vessel are overlaid with an appropriate culture medium and incubated at room temperature.

3. Cell thawing

In the case of subsequent subcultures, the preserved cell culture might have to be used. The water bath is heated to a temperature of 37°C, and the growth media where the cells are to be plated is warmed. The warm medium is added to the culture vessel. The vial with the frozen cells is then placed in the water bath until thawed. After thawing, the via is washed with 70% alcohol on the outside. The cell suspension is pipetted into the cell culture vessel and swirled gently to mix everything. The medium is then incubated overnight under the usual growth conditions. The growth medium is replaced the next day.

4. Trypsin zing Cells

Trypsinization is the method of separating adherent cells from the surface of the culture vessel with the help of proteolytic enzymes. It is done when the cells are to be used for passaging, counting, or other purposes. The medium is removed, and the cells are recovered. The cells are then washed with phosphate buffer. Warm trypsin-EDTA is added to the vessel so as to cover the monolayer. The vessel can be rocked to ensure that the monolayer is coated. The vessel is incubated in a CO_2 incubator at 37°C for 1-3 minutes. The vessel is removed from the incubator, and the flask is firmly tapped on the side with the palm of the hand to assist detachment. Once the cells are dislodged, they are resuspended in an appropriate growth medium containing some amount of serum.

The cells are then separated with the help of syringe needles by disrupting the cell clumps and used accordingly.

The culture media used for animal cell culture are classified as Natural, Artificial, Synthesized. The selection of culture media depends on the objective of experiment and type of cell to be cultured.

Natural Culture Media:

As the name indicates these media are obtained from natural resources like, tissue extracts, biological fluids, plasma clots or coagulants etc.

Blood Plasma:

It provides good nutrition and support to many types of animal cell culture. During sub culturing it provides good protection against traumatic damage and better attachment of cells to glass surfaces. Chicken plasma is most favored for its clarity even on dilution. The plasma is obtained by centrifugation before coagulation. This tissue or cells are placed in such plasma and then coagulation is initiated by addition of thrombin.

Blood Serum:

Blood serum is plasma without fibrinogen.

Blood serum with or without nutritional substances is used as a culture media to grow animal cells. The sera commonly used in animal culture are bovine, horse, and human. Calf and fetal bovine serum are most widely used sera in animal cell culture. Human serum is used sometimes but is needed to be screened for presence of hepatitis and HIV. The composition of a serum is highly complex as it is a mixture of various plasma proteins, peptides, lipids, carbs, enzymes and minerals.

Tissue Extracts:

Commonly used tissue extracts in animal cell culture are, embryo, spleen, liver, bone marrow etc. Chick embryo extract is the most commonly used tissue extract in animal cell culture, it is obtained from 10-12 days old embryos.

Artificial Media:

Synthetic or artificial media are prepared by adding organic or inorganic substances, nutrients, vitamins, proteins, carbs, gaseous phases. Different artificial media are prepared for different types of cells as per their requirement. Some common examples of artificial media are, Minimal Essential Medium (MEM), CMRL 1066, RPMI 1640. Synthetic media re classified as, Serum Containing Media, Serum Free Media.

Serum Containing Media:

It is prepared by **adding 5 to 20 % serum** in serum free medium. Serum is one of the best sources of many basic nutrients, contains hormones, growth factors, proteins, and minerals. Serum **also acts as a buffer.** Serum combines and neutralises many toxins.

Although it's a best source of nutrients it has following disadvantages, Most **expensive** of all ingredients of the culture medium. It **increases difficulties** and cost of downstream processing. Its **content varies** from batch to batch

Serum Free Media:

They are developed to overcome limitations of serum containing media. These media can make t**he medium more selective for particular cell**s as per their requirements e.g. melanocytes can be cultivated in absence of keratinocytes.

As serum is not present there is no problem of toxicity, serum change tests. Bioassays and other processes become easy due to absence of the serum. However, they also have some disadvantages like, Slower growth, Useful only for a few generations. pH control and temperature control required is more. Most media are specific to a particular cell type. Preparation time is more.

Physicochemical Parameters needed for growth animal cell culture:

The temperature of the culture has to be the same as that of the body temperature of the animal from which cells are collected. Osmolarity between 260 m Osm/kg and 320 m Osm/kg is good for many cell lines. Buffers are incorporated for maintaining the pH as per requirement of the cell culture.

Most cell cultures grow well at a pH of 7.4, phenol red is commonly used indicator to detect the pH change in medium. External Carbon dioxide addition is needed for some cell cultures to replenish CO_2 loss. Oxygen is a component of the gas phase as most cells require oxygen for respiration.

Cell damage in the culture is prevented by increasing viscosity of the medium by addition of CMC or PVP. Balanced Salt Solution (BSS) is used as a diluent for vitamins, amino acids to make complete media.

Applications of Animal cell culture

The following are some of the applications of animal cell culture;

a. Production of vaccines

Animal cell culture is an important technique used for the development of viral vaccine production. The technique has been used for the development of a recombinant vaccine against hepatitis B and poliovirus. Immortalized cell lines are used for the large-scale or industrial production of viral vaccines.

b. Recombinant proteins

Animal cell cultures can also be used for the production of recombinant therapeutic proteins like cytokines, hematopoietic growth factors, growth factors, hormones, blood products, and enzymes. Some of the common animal cell lines used for the production of these proteins are baby hamster kidney and CHO cells.

c. Gene Therapy

The development of animal cell culture is critical for the advances in gene therapy. Cells with faulty genes can be replaced by a functional gene in order to remove such defects and diseases.

d. Model systems

Cells obtained from cell culture can be studied as a model system for studies related to cell biology, host-pathogen interactions, effects of drugs, and effects due to changes in the cell composition.

e. Cancer Research

Animal cell culture can be used to study the differences in cancer cells and normal cells as cancer cells can also be cultured. he differences allow more detailed studies on the potential causes and effects of different carcinogenic substances. Normal cells can be culture to form cancer cells by the use of certain chemicals, viruses, and radiation. Cancer cells can also be used as test systems for studies related to the efficiencies of drugs and techniques used in cancer treatment.

f. Production of Biopesticides

Animal cell lines like Sf21 and Sf9 can be used for the production of biopesticides due to their faster growth rate and higher cell density. Organisms like baculovirus can be produced through animal cell culture as well.

www.ingramcontent.com/pod-product-compliance
Lightning Source LLC
Chambersburg PA
CBHW071224230926
51849CB00001B/23
* 9 7 8 9 3 4 8 7 3 4 1 2 9 *